Practical Cultural Psychiatry

Practical Cultural Psychiatry

Dinesh Bhugra
Emeritus Professor of Mental Health and Cultural Diversity
Centre for Affective Disorders
King's College London, UK

Antonio Ventriglio
Department of Mental Health
University of Foggia
Foggia, Italy

Kamaldeep S. Bhui
Professor of Cultural Psychiatry and Epidemiology
Centre Lead for Psychiatry, Wolfson Institute
of Preventive Medicine
Barts and The London School of Medicine and Dentistry
University of London, UK

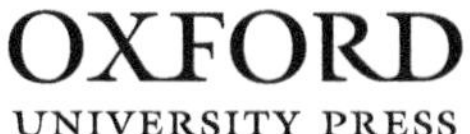

OXFORD
UNIVERSITY PRESS

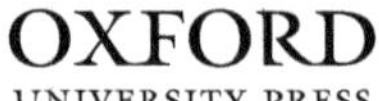

OXFORD
UNIVERSITY PRESS

Great Clarendon Street, Oxford, OX2 6DP,
United Kingdom

Oxford University Press is a department of the University of Oxford.
It furthers the University's objective of excellence in research, scholarship,
and education by publishing worldwide. Oxford is a registered trade mark of
Oxford University Press in the UK and in certain other countries

Published in the United States of America by Oxford University Press
198 Madison Avenue, New York, NY 10016, United States of America

British Library Cataloguing in Publication Data
Data available

Library of Congress Control Number: 2018941857

ISBN 978–0–19–872319–6

Dedicated to Sir David Goldberg—a great teacher, superb
researcher, and dedicated clinician

Preface

In the past decade, cultural psychiatry has come into its own. From our understanding of the impact of cultural factors on causation, expression, and management of mental illness to development and acceptance of cultural formulation in DSM-5, it has become evident that cultures play a major role not only in the genesis but also in the management of psychiatric symptoms. Increasingly, emphasis in teaching and training mental health professionals is on placing the patient at the centre of the consultation and engagement but within the context of their culture. Similarly, the clinician's personal and professional cultures play a role in reaching a diagnosis, and clarify therapeutic strategies, including pharmacological and psychotherapeutic interventions. Micro-identities (which may form part of cultural heritage, including religion) have become much more important in understanding patient experiences. Similarly, cultures dictate accessibility and availability of resources, which will determine who is approached first in determining pathways into care.

In this book, we offer practical aspects of practising cultural psychiatry. From assessment of cultural factors to implementation of pharmacological treatments and various types of psychotherapy, we propose that cultural competence is good clinical practice, and every clinician needs to be aware of the impact culture can have on engagement and therapeutic alliance of patients.

We would like to thank Pete Stevenson, Lauren Tiley, and Rachel Goldsworthy at Oxford University Press for all their hard work and support in seeing the project through.

D.B.
A.V.
K.B.

Contents

Chapter 1

Cultures and their roles: An overview

Introduction

Every individual, no matter where in the world, is born into a culture, grows up in a culture, lives, functions, and dies in a culture. Culture develops and modifies our 'world view'—the way we see the world but, more importantly, perhaps the way we see the world seeing us. The impact of culture is on our attitudes, behaviours, norms, and the way we interact with each other. Within our broad cultural identity, each of us possesses a number of microidentities. Culture is an integral part of our existence, our functioning, and our behaviours. We are born into a cultural context that evolves and is continuously changing, and not born with a fixed culture. We acquire various characteristics because of the cultures in which we grow up and live. Some ingrained cultural characteristics of groups and thus individuals are difficult to change, whereas others alter according to a number of influences. When group or individual cultures change, they undergo a process called acculturation, involving taking up new views and behaviours and giving up older ones; thus this process leads to changes of values, attitudes, and behaviours. The impact of cultural beliefs and behaviours on our bodies, dietary habits, and ability to respond to the demands of life are particularly important in psychiatry.

Definitions

Culture is defined as 'that complex whole which includes knowledge, belief, art, law, morals, custom and any other capabilities and habits acquired by man as a member of society' (Tylor, 1871, p. 1). This definition provides an overview of what is understood by the term culture and the totality of experience. It also emphasizes that we acquire culture; we are born *into* a culture and not *with* a culture. Kirmayer (2018) reminds us that culture has three broad but distinct uses—from the original meaning of cultivation to include standards of refinement and conduct. The second broad meaning is to do with cultural identity and the third as a way of life, including the values, customs, beliefs, and knowledge, as well as the institutions and practices. Kirmayer provides a fuller account of the history of cultural psychiatry.

Interestingly, all these definitions of culture also emphasize that culture is acquired and forms an overall global experience, a 'world view', a way of seeing and making sense of the world. Culture has various aspects, which can be changed through exposure to other cultures, peoples, technologies, and beliefs. Culture is described by Franz Boas as the manifestations of social habits of a community, thus confirming that society and cultures go hand in hand. He goes on to note that the reactions of an individual are affected or shaped by the habits of those belonging to the same cultural group as the individual and those in close proximity (Boas, 1982). These observations are pertinent in our understanding of the way that the members of any culture see themselves and one another, but also how they see others from different cultures and backgrounds. Cultures provide a degree of historical account of the cultural group, as well as values of the individual and give meaning to actions. Patterns of behaviour and patterns for behaviour are influenced by cultures, leading to both subjective and objective world views. Cultural values associated with behaviours, attitudes, and consumption patterns are imbibed subtly and absorbed often without recognizing these.

Kroeber and Kluckhohn (1952) noted 164 definitions of culture but concluded that at the core of these definitions lie diverse patterns of behaviour, which are both implicit and explicit. These behaviours are acquired (as well as transmitted) through symbols that then go on to carry specific meanings. Furthermore, these behaviours carry both historically *acquired* and *selected* (italics added) ideas, which inevitably carry values with them. These values, as well as behaviours, may well be products of favoured and more successful ways of living and succeeding in society certain actions (Kroeber and Kluckhohn, 1952, p. 357). Thus, patterns of behaviour, their symbols, and their meanings become relevant in our understanding of culture. Furthermore, culture should be seen as an intervening variable between human organism and environment (Kroeber and Kluckhohn, 1952, pp. 367–368).

Hsu (1985) uses a multilayered concentric model to describe the relationship between the individual and culture. At the core of the model lies the unconscious, and the outer two layers indicate society and culture. The model thus very clearly emphasizes the interaction between the individual and the society. The role of the individual's personality and the resulting interaction with culture is often not understood properly. The field of anthropology frequently focuses on the broad definitions of culture, and the interaction between culture and the individual personality, or specifically between the society more generally, including its structures and political institutions, and cultural beliefs and behaviours of individuals and groups. The *Diagnostic and Statistical Manual of Mental Disorders-5* (DSM-5) (American Psychiatric Association, 2013) defines culture as referring to systems of knowledge, concepts, rules, and practices that are learned and transmitted across generations. Culture includes language, religion, spirituality, family structures, life-cycle stages, ceremonial rituals, and customs, as well as moral and legal systems. Cultures are open dynamic systems that keep undergoing changes, and individuals change with these systems (p. 749).

The Surgeon General's Report in the USA defines culture broadly as a common heritage, set of beliefs, norms, and values (DHSS, 1999). Culture is referred to as the shared attributes of a group. Anthropologists see and define culture as a system of shared meanings. Thus appears a clear distinction between clinical and anthropological definitions. Gaw (2001) illustrates that components of culture include precepts and concepts, propositions between precepts and concepts (whether these are locational, part or whole, or causal), beliefs, value, and operational procedures. These constitute core clinical aspects of culture. Cultures produce an individual's cultural identity and need to be differentiated from ethnicity, which has a narrower focus, with common ancestry and shared historical past and is often a self-definition.

Geertz (1973) sees culture as a web created by human beings and is thus interpretive rather than experiential science (p. 5). However, human beings do influence culture, experience it, and change culture, which in turn changes them. Cultures are dynamic and not static, change, and alter in response to many external and internal factors. Kleinman (1996, p. 16) sees culture as resulting from daily lived experience and activities, communications, rhythms and rituals of community life, and patterning of social relations. The interaction between individual and society, according to Kleinman, places the locus of culture in the interconnections between body and self, families, work settings, networks, and whole communities, etc.

Culture influences our individual and social cognitions and the way we think both individually and collectively. Cultures give us a sense of identity, of value and purpose, as well as a sense of belonging. Therefore, microcultures can also play a significant role in the formulation of behaviour patterns. These microcultures may emerge from place of education, place of work, and play, etc. Culture also provides a set of rules and standards, adherence to which lead to behaviours that lie within the accepted or sanctioned range of behaviours by the larger cultural group (Haviland, 1990). Thus, the definitions of what is deemed and seen as normal and what is deviant and unacceptable are very strongly influenced and determined by cultures. Inevitably, this affects definitions of psychiatric illness, imparting certain importance to our understanding of the role of cultures. Others, such as Goodenough (1961), have argued that cultures set standards that act as guides, acting as well as interpreting the acts of others. This in turn produces behaviours that are what members of that particular cultural group expect of the individuals. Physical reality, social expectations, and social relations affect these standards.

For psychiatric purposes, the sense of identity or 'self' is important. This identity varies dramatically across cultures. Morris (1994) describes the self as strongly influenced and moulded by cultures. He emphasizes that exploration of the self in functioning, self-consciousness, and agency constitutes a sense of personal identity (p. 13). Looking at six different cultures, Morris goes on to propose that Western concepts of the self are more likely to be individualistic, whereas concepts from Eastern cultures indicate more collectivist cultures. It must also be recognized that, because of globalization and rapid urbanization, many cultures around the globe are in a state of flux and transition, meaning that old values and traditions are giving way to new ones and creating a sense of vacancy and confusion especially across generations. Some societies see new ways of coexistence of new and old traditions, in tension and competition, but it is difficult to give up traditions that feel successful, sacred, or cherished. This may be because they help define the cultural group and provide a way of living with meaning. Learning theories of personhood can explain some aspects of the self, but Morris (1994) cautions us that simplistic typologies of the self may gloss over complexities of self-hood (p. 196).

Cultures communicate meaning through symbols and language, within and across generations. This transmissibility carries generational continuity of ideas, precepts, concepts, and values inherent within the framework that the culture provides (Hughes, 1992, p. 7).

The interaction between biological factors (which are largely genetically determined, although on occasion they may be influenced by environmental factors), psychological factors (determined by upbringing, personality, etc.), and cultural factors (linked with social networks, social determinants, etc.) plays out in a number of ways. This relationship between the three key factors plays out in the aetiology and management of psychiatric disorders.

Kirmayer (2018) states that the construct of culture offers one way to conceptualize differences across cultures, allowing the bringing together of concepts of race, ethnicity, and culture. He suggests that, historically, three major sets of concerns have helped to develop cultural psychiatry. These are: universalism or relativism of psychopathology and healing practices, dilemmas and challenges in providing services to culturally diverse populations, and, finally, the role of psychiatric practice in response to cultural

Box 1.1 Essential characteristics of culture

1. Culture is dynamic
2. Culture informs people and people change culture
3. Culture is learned and taught by a number of means
4. Culture explains systems of symbols and meanings
5. Culture can be reproduced
6. Culture includes objective and subjective patterns of human behaviour
7. Culture moulds and forms the 'world view' and cognitions of the individual
8. People carry multiple cultural identities affected by gender, race, education, etc.
9. Culture changes subtly over time although it can change acutely
10. Culture influences cognitive and social development

history and globalization. Therefore, it is helpful to explore and understand what is meant by culture and its impact on individuals.

The essential characteristics of culture are listed in Box 1.1.

It is vital that clinicians take into account the cultural values, beliefs, and attitudes of patients into any therapeutic interaction. Cultural concepts of the person are critical in our understanding of people facing distress. These concepts also influence where help is sought from and once in the healthcare system what they go through. It is almost universal that individuals who may belong to minority groups, whether it is due to their ethnicity, skin colour, race, religion, or sexual orientation, may face discrimination and prejudice from majority groups. In clinical settings, the clinician must be conscious of the experiences related to prejudice that the patients or their families may have gone through.

Racism

Culture also constructs notions of race, which divides human beings into groups in superficial ways such as skin colour, shape of body, face, etc. Racial constructs and their salience have changed over time and vary across societies. Often the construct of race has no clear biological or scientific underpinnings. However, the concept is socially significant as it can lead to racial ideologies and racism, discrimination, and social exclusion. These negative attitudes may well have a strong negative effect on individuals' mental health and functioning (American Psychiatric Association, 2013, p. 749). Biological inheritance, via genetic material, of a physical characteristic or a physical potential or predisposition is often proposed to relate to the concept of race. Race is not particularly useful as a social category, other than it is persistent and provides a way of trying to classify people into the 'in' and 'out' groups. Using race as a variable to indicate superiority—with additional elements of power—is a contributory component of racism and shapes the allocation of resources.

Racism is seen as an ideology/belief, which indicates that superior races 'deserve' privileges, e.g. health and education. Institutional racism reflects an enforcement of racism that may then be maintained by legal, cultural, religious, educational, economic, political, environmental, and military institutions of society. Racism plays a role in the creation of 'the other', which separates peoples into aliens ('out' groups) and the 'in' group. One type of racism is missionary racism, which suggests that one individual or one group of individuals knows about the needs of the subjugated group better than the group itself does. Another form of racism is described as colour blindness, and assumes that all minority patients are alike and that their needs are the same. Therapists and clinicians may carry these attitudes unconsciously. It is important to recognize and deal with unconscious racial bias.

Racism can have significant effects on the process of diagnosis. Due to prejudice and negative attitudes, with or without stereotyping patients, racism can lead to misdiagnosis, overdiagnosis, and underdiagnosis.

Ethnicity, culture, and practice

Ethnicity is defined in DSM-5 as culturally constructed group identity used to define peoples and communities and rooted in geographical settings and origins, common history, language, religion, and other characteristics of the group, which may be seen as distinctive (American Psychiatric Association, 2013, p. 749). In the UK, ethnicity is self-ascribed and the typologies vary widely. Increasing mobility, inter-marriages, and intermixing of cultures will change ethnicities and create multiple identities. Race, on the other hand, has been seen as a biological variant with physical features determining the racial origins of the individual.

Cultures set standards for behaviour. The way behaviour is defined as abnormal or deviant is decided and dictated by cultures. These are then recognized and accepted by the group as a whole, which in turn affect an individual's own behaviour (Harwood, 1981).

Like other professions, psychiatry itself and the practice of clinical psychiatry have their own cultures, and these form the 'opinion' and the world view of the psychiatrist. To complicate matters further, these subcultures are strongly influenced by the place of training and type of training. For example, a psychoanalyst or psychiatrist training in New York will have a very different 'world view' of psychiatry when compared with that of a biological psychiatrist trained in Germany or Russia or China. Furthermore, those trained in one institution in New York may well have very different views, attitudes, and models compared with others. These individual attitudes, personalities, and cognitions will affect their clinical practice. Thus, any individual will carry with them multiple cultural identities by virtue of their gender, age, and social class, and educational and economic status.

Cultural identity defines an individual. Microidentities provide a degree of confirmation of where the individual's world view may be. Some of these microidentities are variable and perhaps functional. Some of the microidentities are related to religion and to gender, both of which can be changed. Other microidentities may also change. For example, a psychiatrist, when ill, may give up the role of the psychiatrist and take up the role of the patient. However, the presentation in the latter identity and role is likely to be very strongly influenced by the former role.

As an individual's world view is affected by a number of factors, their world view may not always match that of the doctor, thereby creating a degree of tension. Individual identities are both influenced by and related to cultural concepts of the individual self. Cultural identity functions at both individual and group levels. Wachter et al. (2015) point out that microidentities may well reflect aspects of the individual that may be seen as discriminatory. Institutional cultures will affect microidentity, as will religion, gender, educational and economic status, and sexual orientation. Identities are also affected by social structures (Burke, 2004, p. 6). Social and individual identities may not always overlap. For example, a gay black female may choose not to come out as gay, but her racial and gender identities will be apparent and she may choose to attend a black female gay group, thus changing the emphasis altogether in that particular setting only. Thus, in clinical settings, clinicians must take broader cultural identities as well as microidentities into account while assessing as well as managing individuals with psychiatric disorders.

In addition to cultural identities, associated explanations for illness and help-seeking also determine pathways into care. Individuals may choose to see shamans, folk healers, or others as their first port-of-call in comparison with others who may prefer to go directly to the professional health sector. This may be influenced by ease of access to the healthcare system and ability to pay. Explanatory models and idioms of distress are strongly affected by cultural values and cultural identities (including microidentities). There is a variety of ways to define and identify a cultural group and often people see themselves as having multiple cultural identities.

Types of culture

Hofstede (1980/2001) has described five dimensions of cultures. It is worth recalling that one broad categorization is culture as egocentric (individualistic) or sociocentric (collectivist). The characteristic differences between the two are set out in Table 1.1.

In addition, Hofstede (1980/2001) has described four other broad dimensions of culture. Although he described these following a study of multinational companies, these dimensions can help us in exploring cultural values. However, ascertaining all these makes it much more complex in clinical settings. These dimensions are masculine/feminine (characteristics illustrated in Box 1.2); how cultures are good at avoiding uncertainty; how close individuals feel to the centre of power; and long-term orientation of the culture. It would appear that, of these five dimensions, two are not only easy to identify—individualism/collectivism and masculine/feminine—but may play a bigger role in formation of the self.

Thus, even if we take into account egocentric/sociocentric and masculine/feminine dimensions, their interactions with microidentities can create

Table 1.1 Differences between egocentric and sociocentric cultures

Egocentric	Sociocentric
Characteristics	
Nuclear family	Extended/joint family
Status orientated	Status predetermined
Weak social links	Strong social links
Choose life partner	Little or no choice
Independent	Interdependent
Individual advance	Group advance
'Modern'	'Traditional'
Examples	
USA, UK, France	India, Pakistan, Nigeria

Box 1.2 Differences between masculine and feminine cultures

Masculine cultures have greater and stronger differentiation between gender roles and child-rearing patterns. Men are expected to be ambitious, strong, and tough. Sympathy is for the strong. Ego-orientation. Girls are allowed to cry but not boys. In schools, performance is seen as important, and a competitive nature is encouraged actively. Public praise. Family is important. Quick marriages. Teachers pay more attention to boys. *Latin American cultures are more masculine.*

In feminine cultures, both genders are expected to be tender and take care of relationships. Both genders should be modest. Lower job stress. Child rearing is shared. Children are treated as equal. More unmarried cohabitation. Children are encouraged and socialized not to be aggressive. *Scandinavian cultures are more feminine.*

complex multilayered interactions affecting therapeutic help-seeking as well as therapeutic alliances. It is worth acknowledging that cultures are not homogenous and therefore not all members of a particular culture will have all the characteristics of that specific culture. Thus, once again, Hsu's (1985) concept of concentric layers comes to the fore.

If the patient carries these multiple dimensions with them, it is inevitable that the clinician will too. Culture as a concept is equally applicable to professionals who treat them and they too have a shared set of beliefs, norms, and values depending upon their own cultural background, age, experience, institutions they trained in, and the institutional cultures within which they work. Any professional group's culture can be gleaned from the jargon they use, the orientation of their learning, and their formed world views.

Individualistic cultures refer to society where the ties between individuals are loose and everyone is expected to look after himself/herself and their immediate family. Collectivist or sociocentric cultures are those where people from birth onwards are integrated into strong cohesive in-groups which, throughout their lifetime, continue to protect them in exchange for unquestioning loyalty. Whereas individualism means I-ness, I-consciousness, autonomy, emotional independence, individual initiative, right to privacy, pleasure-seeking, financial security, and need for specific friendship, collectivism refers to We-ness, We-consciousness, collective identity, emotional interdependence, group solidarity, sharing duties and obligations, need for stable and predetermined friendships, and group decisions (Hofstede, 1980/2001). In egocentric cultures, individuals choose and the choices mostly are rational, discreet, autonomous, and self-sufficient, and individuals are respectful of the rights of others. The identity in egocentric settings may well be confined by achievement. Sociocentric or collectivist settings focus on common good and individuals are bound by relationships; needs of others are put before one's own needs, and justice and institutions are seen as an extension of the kinship and family, which may well be seen as interconnectedness, indicating that systems can be manipulated. There may be elements of paternalism. From a migration perspective, individuals from egocentric cultures are good at entering and leaving new social groups. Egocentric individuals are also better at forming in-groups and, at least superficially, appear more sociable. It makes sense that egocentric individuals, whether they are from sociocentric societies or from egocentric societies, will settle better in egocentric societies. Sociocentric individuals from sociocentric societies may settle better in egocentric societies, especially if they have individuals with similar cultural values; otherwise they will feel alienated and isolated and thus will find it difficult to settle down.

Masculinity stands for a society to which social gender roles are clearly distinct. Men are supposed to be assertive, tough, and focused on material success, whereas women are expected to be more modest, tender, and concerned with quality of life (Hofstede, 2001, p. 297). He goes on to describe femininity as standing for society in which social gender roles overlap, and both men and women are supposed to be modest, tender, and concerned with quality of life. The gender role patterns in families are affected by social and cultural expectations.

Migrants/refugees/asylum-seekers

The number of people migrating for economic/educational or political reasons is rising across the globe. However, in many countries there seems to be some confusion between migration, refuge, and asylum, and all three categories are treated in the same way. Refugees and asylum-seekers are both defined legally.

Stages of migrations have been identified as pre-migration, migration and post-migration (Bhugra, 2004). These stages may not always be clear-cut and may run into each other and show considerable overlap. The periods of pre-migration and migration may also vary dramatically depending upon the purpose of migration, timing and preparations. Figure 1.1 shows the stages and areas to assess that may affect mental health. Duration of post-migration adjustment may last a long time, perhaps even across generations,

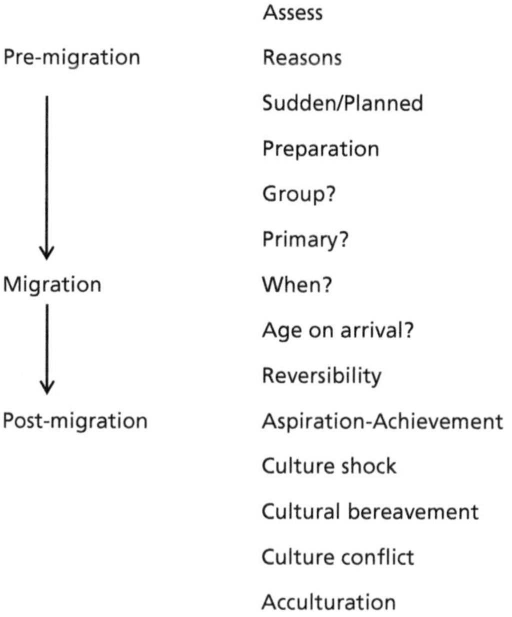

Figure 1.1 Stages of migration.

although there are very few studies looking at acculturation in third-generation migrants.

Migrants, refugees, and asylum-seekers may face specific issues related to the actual act of migration and post-migration phase. Eisenbruch (1990, 1991) has described the notions of cultural bereavement experienced by refugees. Cultural bereavement is seen because of experiencing loss of social structures, cultural values, and (cultural) identity, and is highlighted by an almost unnatural attachment to the past. This may also be considered as idealization of the past and seeing the culture left behind as perfect and ideal. There is the question of whether those who migrate for economic and educational reasons also experience cultural bereavement. The 'odd' experiences described by refugees included feeling guilty (at their own survival, at their abandonment of other loved ones or families), intrusive thoughts and images of their elders and their own past, and morbid thoughts along with anger. Perceived locus of control in managing this grief and expression of grief will both play an important role in the development of cultural bereavement. Western constructs on bereavement may have only a limited value in explaining expressions of grief and its management in other cultures

(Bhugra and Becker, 2005). It seems highly likely that cultural loss and abandonment may produce feelings of cultural bereavement. Individuals' personalities will influence their response to migration. In addition, whether they migrated alone or as part of a group will also play a role in the genesis and coping with cultural bereavement.

Another response to migration is 'culture shock'. This term is used to explain the shock experienced by some migrants after their move to the new culture (Oberg, 1960). Culture shock affects various aspects of an individual's functioning where, perhaps related to loss and subsequent stress, alienation related to the new culture may set in. Resulting anxiety and feelings of helplessness and impotence may confirm their feelings that the new culture is not only remarkably different, but also unwelcoming and alien. This alienation may produce further anxiety in the individual. Another possible reaction to migration is the notion of culture conflict, which relates to a degree of conflict between two members of the same culture, but often across generations or across cultures too, e.g. that of the migrant and the new culture. Aspects of an individual's cultural identity may well become more rigid in the context of the migration experiences. On the other hand, those born and brought up in the new culture may hold values of the new society, and this tension may lead to culture conflict. It may also occur between one culture and the broader culture. Culture conflict is an affective and cognitive dissonance and may result from attempts to assimilate values of the new culture; it reflects dilemmas experienced by the individual in trying to integrate the two opposing views. Culture conflict has been used to explain some of the high rates of some psychiatric disorders experienced by some ethnic minority groups (Bhugra, 2004).

It is possible that, when individuals migrate, they may not always go through all stages of migration or these stages may well merge into one another. It is also worth remembering that not all minority ethnic groups belong to a migrant group, as it may have occurred generations previously. Migrants may migrate for any number of reasons, whereas refugees and asylum-seekers may well move because of political, sexual orientation, or religious persecution. Individuals may migrate singly or in groups, thereby losing their social networks or carrying these with them to wherever they move.

Cultural (including language) differences between country of origin and country of migration may be minimal or extreme. Thus, adjustment may well be easy or very difficult. For example, differences in religion, dietary habits, language, dress, etc. may cause further difficulties for migrants and how they settle in the new setting. In addition, depending upon their educational, social, and economic status they may be welcomed or

> ## Box 1.3 Assessment of acculturation
>
> Assess in broad areas:
> 1. Language—its practice, e.g. spoken only at home, only at work, or elsewhere
> 2. Cognitive style
> 3. Personality traits, including attitudes
> 4. Individual identity
> 5. Acculturative stress
> 6. Religion—its practice
> 7. Attitudes and changes
>
> These must be measured across the individual's cultural group as well as that of the majority group.

they may feel further alienated. In some circumstances, migrants may go through a process of adjustment where they may have to learn to deal with discrepancy between their aspirations and their achievements. They may have migrated with the view that they will achieve a lot more than they succeed in doing in different fields such as employment, education, housing, etc.

Adjustment to migration will influence the process of acculturation and may well reduce the likelihood of culture conflict with the majority culture. However, equally importantly, culture conflict may emerge between two generations of the migrant culture. The assessment of cultural identity is similar to that of acculturation (Box 1.3). Various areas of cultural identity will need to be explored.

Acculturation

Acculturation is the process initiated by two or more cultures that encounter each other either directly or indirectly on a prolonged or short-term basis. Acculturation deals with the cultural and psychological change that an individual experiences following contact between cultural groups and individual members (Redfield et al., 1936). Such contact and change may well result from direct or indirect contact between cultures. The former may be due to colonization, occupation, or migration, whereas the latter may be through print and social media, television, and cinema. Acculturation is the process through which individuals or groups of individuals may acquire the attitudes of other groups and, by sharing their experiences, may develop bicultural or monocultural responses.

In addition, Berry (1970, 1997) argues that acculturation must look into how ethnocultural groups and individuals relate to each other and change as a response to two cultures coming together. Acculturation and identity are strongly interlinked. In the first instance, individuals may well have to deal with two cultures with some tension between the two ways of living and looking at the world. Berry (2007) emphasizes that not all groups and individuals go through the same process of acculturation. These acculturative strategies (Berry, 1980, 2003) are used in varying ways depending upon a plethora of antecedent factors.

Four acculturation strategies and responses have been described by Berry (1970, 1997, 2007, 2018). These must be seen in the context of both individual and group settings. Furthermore, acculturative strategies also bring about change in attitudes and behaviours towards their own culture. Ethnocultural groups may use strategies related to integration, separation, assimilation, and marginalization. Berry (2007, 2018) highlights that there are five stages over time, which include exposure to acculturation as a life event that may produce stress, thereafter developing coping strategies and stress, and in the end it may lead to adaptation. Adaptations may be sociocultural or psychological.

Acculturation processes involve cultural identification, cultural, structural, moral, civic, and behavioural (whether they encounter prejudice or no prejudice) changes. Response of the new country will also determine what stages individuals go through and how the individuals as well as those around them manage these stages. Berry (2007, 2018) suggests that the new country may develop different identities as a country, such as multiculturalism, melting pot, or exclusion or segregation. Acculturation can lead to integration, separation, assimilation, and marginalization. Assessment of acculturation is shown in Box 1.3. Family set-up, employment, diet, leisure activities, attitudes, and specific behaviours may need to be assessed.

Assimilation

This is the process of adjustment when two cultures (one to which the individual belongs and the other to which they may have migrated) lead to the individual acquiring the attitudes of the new culture and gaining historical perspective and sharing of experiences. This may lead the individual to be absorbed into the majority culture and they may lose subtle cultural nuances of their own culture. Assimilation could be seen as a one-way process.

Biculturalism

Some groups and individuals are well placed in moving across two or more cultures and feeling very comfortable in each. They may be equally fluent in two languages and easily move between them. It is helpful to assess whether an individual speaks the new language everywhere or only in the place of employment. Similarly, one should note whether they wear cultural symbols or clothes on specific occasions or everywhere, thereby giving a clue to the degree of acculturation. This denotes the degree of comfort across both cultures.

Deculturation

Deculturation often occurs when, due to war, one culture invades another and the subjugated groups are stripped of their cultures, as was observed with aboriginal groups and during apartheid periods. Dressler (2007, 2018) points out that cultural consonance plays an important role. Cultural consonance allows an understanding of collective meanings attributed to illness experiences. As culture is both learned and shared and the locus of culture is both within the individual and in the social group, Dressler (2007, 2018) goes on to suggest that cultural consonance is cognitive as well as understanding of sharing of culture within the larger group. Cultural consonance is about linked collective cultural values as well as individual ones and can affect patient outcomes.

Minority groups

Minority groups, whether they are migrant groups or not, may have special needs in terms of explaining their distress and seeking help. They may hesitate in seeking help due to stigma and may feel that the clinicians from the majority culture may not understand or misunderstand their language, their attitudes, and the importance of their rituals, behaviours, and explanatory models. There may also be generational differences in help-seeking. Younger generations may well have similar models and attitudes as well as expectations from therapeutic encounters as those of the majority culture, whereas older individuals or migrants may retain their original cultural values, expectations, and attitudes.

Cultural competence

Cultural competence in essence is basic good clinical practice where the clinician sees patients in the context of the patient's culture as well as their own personal cultural values and prejudices. Often it is erroneously assumed that only minority patients have cultures. Cultural competence is defined as an ability to understand and be aware of cultural factors in the therapeutic interaction between the therapist and the patient. These include awareness of social, cultural, religious factors, attitudes, behaviours, models, and explanations. This should be applicable to all patients and all therapeutic interactions. Cultural competency constitutes cultural sensitivity, cultural empathy, and cultural insight. Cultural competence should be considered at both the individual/clinical level as well as at the institutional level. It is possible that even when individuals are being sensitive the institutions may carry unconscious cultural biases in not providing access to appropriate food, cosmetic products, etc. The cultural knowledge, cultural skills, and cultural attitudes of the patient should be explored by the clinician in a culturally sensitive and culturally appropriate environment. Training for clinicians as well as support staff in managing unconscious bias may help. Using cultural mediators or cultural brokers may provide a useful tool for increasing cultural competence. Cultural competence is to be seen as the clinician being not only culturally aware but also being culturally knowledgeable, culturally sensitive, and skilled to deliver culturally appropriate and relevant interventions. A culturally competent clinician will be able to engage patients and their families and carers, and will be able to provide a culturally relevant assessment and interventions. Such clinicians will also be aware of their own cultural biases and prejudices. As a result the patients and their families will feel better equipped to engage in therapeutic alliance.

Patient interviews

Irrespective of ethnicity, each patient carries culture and cultural values with them that affect their help-seeking and therapeutic adherence and alliance. These models are related to how they see their distress—whether it is physical, psychological, social, or a mix of these. In many cultures, explanatory models will include natural or supernatural models.

Patients and their carers may be more interested in understanding why something has gone wrong and potential interventions. Clinicians may be interested in what is wrong, and this discrepancy needs to be handled carefully. Where the interaction takes place will bring with it certain issues that need to be taken into account. For example, home assessments will carry

Box 1.4 LEARN

Listen to the patient and their informants
Explain your reasons for asking questions
Acknowledge the patient's/family's/carer's concerns
Recommend a course of action using a biopsychosocial model
Negotiate a plan for therapeutic engagement and alliance

Source data from *Western Journal of Medicine*, 12, Berlin EA and Fowkes WC, A teaching framework for cross-cultural healthcare: application in family practice, pp. 93–98, 1983.

different weight than a hospital assessment or assessment in a police station or prison setting.

There are basic principles that must be remembered when assessing patients, and these are illustrated by using the examples of two strategies. The first of these is LEARN, which provides a framework for interviewing patients. LEARN is illustrated in Box 1.4. Within this model, it is essential that patients' cultural values are included at every stage. The clinician needs to feel comfortable in asking the questions related to cultural values no matter how bizarre these may appear.

The second model illustrated here is described by Rust et al. (2006), providing a CRASH course in cultural competence, shown in Box 1.5. This approach sets out some key components of culturally competent healthcare. These authors suggest cultural awareness on the part of the individual clinician and also sensitivity and humility as part of cultural competence.

Cultural competence is further detailed in Chapter 2 (see Box 2.1), along with an understanding of cultural formulation (see Chapter 4).

Box 1.5 CRASH

Consider culture at all levels of assessment
Respect for patients and their values
Assess differences with therapist and with culture
Sensitivity/self-awareness
Humility

Ethnicity & Disease © 2006. Rust G et al. Published by ISHIB. Adapted with permission. All rights reserved.

The core message is that, in spite of their status, all patients have cultural values and aspects to their understanding and help-seeking. Therefore, all clinicians need to take on board cultural sensitivity, cultural knowledge, and cultural understanding as well as cultural differences, which may be colouring their own responses.

Conclusions

Every individual has culture and every clinician does too. These cultural values are part of the core identity of the individual and that of the profession. These influence both cultural identities and multiple microidentities. Clinicians have their own language and their own cultures, and sometimes the interaction between the clinician and the patient may become confrontational if clinicians choose not to take cultural factors and cultural nuances into account. Cultural competence is simply good clinical practice. Awareness of cultural values and cultural knowledge and cultural sensitivity are important aspects of clinical encounters.

References

American Psychiatric Association. (2014). *Diagnostic and Statistical Manual of Mental Disorders*, 5th edn. Washington DC: APA.

Berlin EA, Fowkes WC (1983). A teaching framework for cross-cultural healthcare: application in family practice. *West J Med*, **12**, 93–98.

Berry JW (1970). Marginality, stress and ethnic identification in an acculturated Aboriginal community. *J Cross Cult Psychol*, **1**, 239–252.

Berry JW (1980). Acculturation as varieties of adaptation. In Padilla A (ed). *Acculturation: Theories, models and findings*. Boulder, CO: Westview, pp. 9–25.

Berry JW (1997). Immigration, acculturation and adaptation. *Appl Psychol: an international review*, **46**, 5–68.

Berry JW (2003). Conceptual approaches to acculturation. In Chun E, Bals-Organista P, Marin G (eds). *Acculturation*. Washington, DC: American Psychological Association, pp. 17–37.

Berry JW (2007). Acculturation and identity. In Bhugra D, Bhui K (eds). *Textbook of Cultural Psychiatry*. Cambridge: Cambridge University Press, pp. 169–178.

Berry JW (2018). Acculturation and identity. In Bhugra D, Bhui K (eds). *Textbook of Cultural Psychiatry*, 2nd edn. Cambridge: Cambridge University Press, pp. 185–193.

Bhugra D (2004). Migration and mental health. *Acta Psych Scand*, **109**(4), 243–258.

Bhugra D, Becker M (2005). Migration, cultural bereavement and cultural identity. *World Psych*, **4**(1), 18–24.

Boas F (1982). Summary of the work of the committee in British Columbia. In Stocking GW (ed.). *A Franz Boas Reader: The Shaping of American Anthropology 1883–1911*. Chicago: University of Chicago Press, pp. 801–893.

Burke PJ (2004). Identities and social structures. *Social Psychol Quart*, **67**, 5–15.

DHHS. (1999). U.S. Department of Health and Human Services. Mental Health: A report of the Surgeon General. Rockville, MD. Also see U.S. Department of Health and Human Services. (2001). Mental Health: Culture, Race, and Ethnicity—A Supplement to Mental Health: A Report of the Surgeon General. Rockville, MD: U.S. Department of Health and Human Services, Substance Abuse and Mental Health Services Administration, Center for Mental Health Services.

Dressler WW (2007). Cultural consonance. In Bhugra D, Bhui K (eds). *Textbook of Cultural Psychiatry*. Cambridge: Cambridge University Press, pp. 179–190.

Dressler WW (2018). Cultural consonance. In Bhugra D, Bhui K (eds). *Textbook of Cultural Psychiatry*, 2nd edn. Cambridge: Cambridge University Press, pp. 194–203.

Eisenbruch M (1990). Cultural bereavement interview: a new clinical approach for refugees. *Psych Clin N Am*, **13**, 715–735.

Eisenbruch M (1991). From post-traumatic stress disorder to cultural bereavement: diagnosis of Southeast Asian refugees. *Soc Sci Med*, **33**, 673–680.

Gaw AC (2001). *Cross-Cultural Psychiatry*. Washington, DC: American Psychiatric Publishing.

Geertz C (1973). *The Interpretation of Cultures*. New York: Basic Books.

Goodenough WH (1961). Comments as cultural revolution. *Daedalus*, **90**, 521–528.

Harwood A (1981). (ed.). *Ethnicity and Medical Care*. Cambridge, MA: Harvard University Press.

Haviland WA (1990). *Cultural Anthropology*. New York: Holt, Rhinehart & Winston.

Hofstede G (1980/2001). *Culture's Consequences*. Thousand Oaks, CA: Sage.

Hsu FLK (1985). The self in cross-cultural perspective. In Marsella A, Hsu FK and DeVos F (eds). *The Self in a Cross-Cultural Perspective*. New York: Tavistock, pp. 24–55.

Hughes CC (1992). Culture in clinical psychiatry. In: Gaw AC (ed.). *Culture, Ethnicity and Mental Illness*. Washington DC: American Psychiatric Press, pp. 1–41.

Kirmayer L (2018). Cultural psychiatry in historical perspective. In Bhugra D, Bhui K (eds). *Textbook of Cultural Psychiatry*, 2nd edn. Cambridge: Cambridge University Press, pp. 1–17.

Kleinman A (1996). How is culture important for DSM-IV. In Mezzich J et al. (eds). *Culture and Psychiatric Diagnosis*. Washington DC: American Psychiatric Press, pp. 15–25.

Kroeber AL, Kluckhohn C (1952). *Culture: A critical review of concepts and definitions*. Papers of the Peabody Museum of American Archaeology & Ethnology. Cambridge, MA: Harvard University Museum.

Morris B (1994). *Anthropology of the Self: The individual in cultural perspective*. London: Pluto Press.

Oberg K (1960). Culture shock: adjustment to new cultural environments. *Pract Anthrop*, **7**, 177–182.

Redfield R, Linton R, Herskovits MJ (1936). Memorandum on the study of acculturation. *Am Anthrop*, **38**(1), 149–152.

Rust G, Kondwani K, Martinez R, et al. (2006). A crash-course in cultural competence. *Ethn Dis*, **16**(2 Suppl 3): S3–36.

Tylor E (1871). *Primitive Culture* (vol. 1). London: John Murray.

Wachter M, Ventriglio A, Bhugra D (2015). Micro-identities, adjustment and stigma. *Int J Soc Psych*, **61**(5), 436–437.

Chapter 2

Therapeutic encounters

Introduction

When individuals are feeling unwell and they identify their odd behaviour or mood or abnormal thoughts as distressing or confusing, they may consult their family members and others around them to make sense of their experience. People around the individual may see this as pathology that may require intervention. In the first instance, they may choose to deal with the symptoms by themselves. They may discuss with others and seek advice in the personal, folk, or social sectors. If these approaches do not help, they may seek advice from one or more health professionals. In many settings, the first port of call is likely to be the primary care physician, who may choose to treat individuals or may refer them to secondary care. These steps and decisions depend upon the available resources and the healthcare models being practised in that particular culture. In addition, how the individual and those around them see the causes of this distress will influence where they go and how pathways into care are followed.

Cultural factors interact with the past and previous experiences of individuals and help mould the presentation and help-seeking patterns. Race, gender, religion, sexual orientation, culture itself, education, social, and economic factors will all play a role in the way that distress is understood, expressed, and help sought. In psychiatric practice, it is vital that clinicians understand aspects of culture that may be contributing to the precipitation, presentation, and perpetuation of psychiatric disorders. Cultural beliefs, attitudes, and values of the patient and those of the doctor, along with those of the institution, are probably different and may lead to conflict. Hence, it behoves clinicians and managers alike to ensure that the patient's cultural values are taken into account in the planning and delivery of psychiatric services. As discussed in Chapter 1, it must be remembered that cultures are dynamic and change subtly over time, or they may change acutely so that the clinician is aware of potential confusion.

Culture and illness

It is important and helpful to recognize that, once individuals experience distress and identify it as such, it does not turn them into patients. How patients experience, interpret, and explain their distress and where, when, and how they seek help is part of the illness behaviour. This illness behaviour is strongly influenced by cultural factors and norms. How they understand what they are going through and how they express their experiences all contribute to their illness behaviour. Different cultural groups see normal and abnormal (whether it is physical or mental or a mixture of the two) in different ways. Individuals may have causal explanations about their illness experiences and these may well include supernatural, natural, psychological, social, and medical explanations, or a combination of these. Supernatural explanations include beliefs about the evil eye, djinns, or experiences of possession, soul loss, and breach of taboos and affront to ancestor spirits. Natural explanations may include disharmony of elements in the body or outside, noxious environments, microsystem changes, etc. Somatomedical explanations will include dysfunction of organs or systems, physiological imbalance, and insufficient vitality (Tseng and Streltzer, 2008). These authors go on to contrast folk/faith/traditional health practices with allopathic practices, and argue that the former groups are more interested in the whole individual than just the symptom. Furthermore, these medical systems antedate modern medicine and, in places where the access to medical care may be limited, they may be preferred as the first port of call. Shields et al. (2016) have illustrated an interesting example of faith healers and modern psychiatry working together. These authors reported from Western India, where an innovative collaborative programme at a *dargah* (Muslim holy place where people with mental illness go to pray) was developed. Over a period of 2 years or so, medical practitioners worked with faith healers and, through dialogue and collaboration, developed programmes to establish a shared role for care and recovery of persons with mental illness. The medical professionals assessed patients with mental illness and worked with faith healers to encourage better compliance. Despite differing practices, a close collaboration between faith-based and allopathic mental health practitioners was encouraged and established.

Disease versus illness

Although semantically meaning the same experience, disease and illness reflect different things to anthropologists and medical practitioners. Disease is literally dis-ease, and physicians are trained to diagnose and treat diseases—that is what they are interested in because disease represents pathology. Hence, disease is considered objectively and universally similar in nature. Tseng and Streltzer (2008) suggest that disease should be seen as the medical definition of sickness by professionals, and can be explained by physiological or biological/structural (pathological) changes that can explain the alterations in functioning of the individual. In contrast, illness refers to the patient's psychological construct of the perceptions, experiences, and understanding of the suffering (Tseng and Streltzer, 2008). Illness may have to be hidden from others because it affects an individual's social functioning as well as their social status and social standing. Patients 'suffer' from illnesses, which are experiences of disvalued changes in states of being and in social functioning (Eisenberg, 1977). Disease is the concept used by professionals. On the other hand, individuals who may be going through distressing experiences use illness to describe their experiences. Eisenberg (1977) notes that shifting patterns of symptoms among military neuro-psychiatric casualties illustrate the shaping of response to stress by culture, which channels overt expression into explicit syndromes of illness. There is a discrepancy between dis-ease as it is conceptualized by the physician and the illness as experienced by the patient, which is likely to affect therapeutic adherence and alliance. Often patients are interested in social functioning and they may be able to manage their symptoms as long as they can carry out their expected functions. Thus, from the beginning of the therapeutic interaction there is a disjunction between the doctor and the individual, who 'becomes' a patient. The term sickness in many parts of the world is defined by society to regulate sick behaviours, like sick leave, sickness benefits, etc. Clinicians must understand these differences and take them on board if they are to engage patients successfully. The tension between the two aspects of the same experience is clear, and requires understanding and managing irrespective of cultural values, even though cultures will affect these experiences and their underlying explanations.

Doctor–patient interaction

Therapeutic adherence depends upon the alliance between the patient and the doctor, and reasons for this success are many. These include the experience of the clinician in engagement of the patient after understanding the needs and expectations of the patients. On the other hand, patients' expectations of the therapeutic encounter will influence their engagement, especially if their expectations are met. Patients often have different expectations of the outcomes from the clinical interaction, and these are strongly influenced by cultural values and how the role of clinician is seen. The clinician–patient interaction is at the core of the therapeutic encounter and forms the basis of therapeutic alliance. There is no doubt that the culture of the patient, the culture of the clinician, and the culture of the healthcare system, as well as that of the institution within which the therapeutic encounter takes place are all important aspects in not only clinical care delivery but also engagement of the patients, their carers, and families; therefore these all influence outcomes. The doctor–patient relationship has to be collaborative and the patient has to have faith in the doctor to take the treatment and adhere to it. The doctor has a professional responsibility to be empathic, caring, and understanding when working with patients, as well as their families and carers. In cultures that are authoritative, traditional, or sociocentric, the doctor may have more power or may be seen as having more power and influence. Such a power differential in psychiatric care will play a major role in therapeutic engagement and compliance.

Cultural factors determine the idioms that are used to express distress, and will be influenced by basic understanding of the symptoms and their importance in social functioning. Cultures may well define clinical need and help-seeking. In many cultures, mental illness is attributed to supernatural causative factors, which means that the individuals may be encouraged to seek help from faith healers. Societies and cultures define deviance and abnormality, which indicates the sources of help-seeking and pathways into care. The basic primary aim of the patient's interaction with the doctor is to attain relief or amelioration of symptoms, very often because they want to get better and get on with their lives, to look after their families and others. Doctors may be interested in reaching a diagnosis whereas the patient may want to understand what is causing their distress and what is to be done about it so that they can get back to better social functioning.

The main purpose of the doctor–patient interaction depends upon the ability of the clinician to establish a relationship that will allow the patient to feel comforted. Clinicians may choose to lead the consultation so that they can develop an understanding of the patient's distress and symptoms.

When the patient and the doctor are from different cultures, the doctor must attempt to explore cultural similarities as well as differences. Even if the person seeking help and the clinician are from the same cultural background, it is entirely possible that microidentities and different cultural facets will cause unnecessary and unacceptable tension. It is imperative that the clinician manages ethnicity/race/culturally related transference as well as countertransference. The interaction often starts from a disproportionate imbalance of power. In many cultures, doctors are seen to hold power of life and death, so patients and their families and carers may well hand over the responsibility of their care totally to them, whereas in other cultures patients may expect equal involvement in any decision-making. These days often patients present to the clinician with print-outs from the internet about their condition, medication, and its side effects and other information.

Box 2.1 gives a basic framework for cultural aspects of basic clinical assessment. Such assessments must explore personal cultural biases and prejudices on part of the clinician but, equally importantly, that of the patient, who may see this as a sign of openness and acceptance on part of the clinician. In psychiatric assessments, both verbal and non-verbal communication styles are important. Facial expressions and language can prove to be significant in sharing information.

Both verbal and non-verbal communications play a significant role in the totality of expressing distress and explaining what the patient and their families are going through. Therefore, clinical assessment requires attention to not only what is being said but also what remains unexpressed. These expressions and unexpressed ideas and distress will strongly influence assessment and faith in the clinician. Thus, clinicians must be aware of non-verbal communication that patients may use to express their distress and dissatisfaction (see Chapter 3). Inevitably, both verbal and non-verbal communications are strongly influenced by cultures, and these may change because of acculturation. Verbal communication will be affected by the use of language and grasp of subtle nuances in speech, dialect, and slang. If the patient's primary language is different from that of the clinician, then the latter must take into account potential problems and misunderstandings and take steps to avoid these. Prolonged periods of assessment may be necessary for some individuals. It is important that, if interpreters are needed, they are properly

---

Box 2.1 Cultural aspects of the basic assessment

It is critical that, as part of the therapeutic encounter, clinicians are:

(i) Aware of the cultural beliefs of the patient (in the same way as their own) related to culture beliefs, history, heritage, conscious and unconscious biases, prejudices, and values.

(ii) Aware and have knowledge of social structures within the culture, including institutional barriers that an individual patient may face.

(iii) Aware of subtle, overt, and covert ways of communications that are very strongly influenced by culture.

(iv) At the same time, idioms of distress and explanatory models should be explored in a systematic way.

trained in medical interpretation and that clinicians know how to use their skills and competencies; therefore they may require training.

It must be emphasized that in psychiatric settings often the clinical assessment is an ongoing process, as is the clinical engagement. Therefore, the initial contact is about establishing context of help-seeking and understanding the patient's needs and the views of their family and carers. The clinical diagnosis is certainly important, but the clinician should not rush into it. The assessment itself is a collaborative therapeutic event, which should lead to proper therapeutic engagement and subsequent therapeutic relationship.

In many cultures, individuals may choose to keep some physical distance from the clinician, who may be seen as a source of wise advice. Hence, keeping the distance is to be understood in this context and not as a pathology of avoidance.

The clinician, if dealing with patients from other cultures, may need to explore in the consultation some of the very basic cultural factors. These would include the basic cultural values and understanding of racial and ethnic identities. The clinician should also try to explore whether the individual has been exposed to any racial or racist events directly or indirectly, which may well influence the onset of their illness and their attitudes to help-seeking.

Clinical assessment should be set up as outlined in Box 2.2.

Box 2.2 Setting up clinical assessments

1. Be aware of the *purpose* of assessment—whether it is for admission, support, or reports.
2. Be aware of patients' cultural backgrounds, as well as those of their families.
3. Be aware of linguistic needs.
4. Be prepared to work with interpreters.
5. Be prepared to explore the patient's cultural strengths and weaknesses.
6. Confirm whether you have understood the terms patients and their families use.
7. Identify idioms of distress.
8. Identify explanatory models.

Explanatory models

The explanatory model is what individuals make of their distress and experience. This includes a basic understanding of what they see as being the problem in the first place, their explanations of what the actual and perceived causes are, what they think is needed to treat it, and what they foresee the outcome to be.

Weiss (2018) emphasizes that working with explanatory models enables health professionals to evaluate clinical problems based not only on what they know about the medical practice from their professional disciplinary training; this is also informed from the vantage points of the patients and families who are directly affected. Kleinman (1980) describes the explanatory model as notions about an episode of sickness and its treatment that are employed by those engaged in the clinical process. This model is neither static nor singular and may well change in response to a number of factors. The emic and etic framework advanced by Pike (1967) relies on linguistics to describe what is from within (emic) and from outside (etic). This distinction in the early stages also reflected the differences between personal and professional thinking. Weiss (2018) argues that explanatory models are also a statement of theory developed as a product of society's understanding of disease experience. Explanatory models allow personal expression and explanation of mental or physical distress. For example, in India physical symptoms such as joint pains may well be seen as caused by 'gas', which moves around the body, and the treatment therefore must take into account prohibiting foods which may be contributing to increased production of gas.

Standardized questionnaires such as Explanatory Model Interview Catalogue (EMIC; Weiss, 1997) and Short Explanatory Model Interview (SEMI; Lloyd et al., 1998), to name just two, can be utilized to explore explanatory models, but a mixture of qualitative and quantitative assessments may be more helpful.

The main questions that the clinician may ask to explore explanatory models are illustrated in Box 2.3.

The purpose of assessment is to understand the idioms of distress but also the explanatory models held by both the patients and their carers and families. An understanding of these models is critical in establishing goals of treatment and planning the treatment. It is important to remember that the patients and their families are essential partners in planning and accepting treatments.

The doctor–patient interaction is strongly influenced by patients' explanatory models, their idioms of distress (whether these are used and recognized

> ## Box 2.3 Questions that explore explanatory models
>
> - What do you call your problem?
> - What do you think caused your problem?
> - Why do you think it started when it did?
> - What does your illness do to you?
> - What does your illness do to others around you, e.g. family?
> - What does your illness do to your ability to function, to work?
> - How severe is it?
> - How long do you think it is likely to last?
> - What do you fear/worry most about your illness?
> - What do you think will get you better?
> - What will happen if it does not get better?
> - Does it need treatment? If so, what is the best option?
> - What will happen if it is not treated?
>
> Source data from Kleinman A (1980) *Patients and their Healers in the Context of their Cultures*. Berkley, CA: University of California Press.

by the doctor), and what each side expects from the therapeutic encounter. In addition, age, gender, social, economic, and education status will play a role. The doctor's experience and educational status, etc. will also affect the therapeutic interaction (Figure 2.1).

There is no doubt that society and cultures both influence sickness and illness behaviours directly through assimilation and indirectly through access to education and other social factors. There is no doubt that cultures and society dictate where and how healing takes place. This can be illustrated by the fact that treatment options moved from asylums into the community and in many settings assessments and treatments are being offered at home. Society and culture construct a reality within which its members live and function. The practice of medicine, through its cultures and institutions, also creates and constructs a reality that may be different from that of the patient. When the patient and the doctor encounter each other, these two realities interact in both predictable and unpredictable ways.

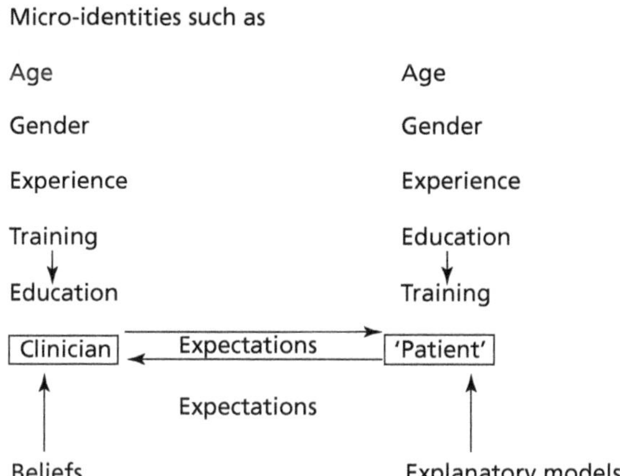

Figure 2.1 The therapeutic encounter.

Culture provides a structure to individuals within which they are born, live, work, and function. Within the medical institutions, the ill individual has to follow the culture of the institution, its rules, and its reality. To complicate matters further, both medicine and society guide the acts of their members and construct medical and social worlds through beliefs and interactions. There is no doubt that the concepts of pathogenesis of psychiatric disorders vary according to societal, cultural, and personal beliefs. Patients, their carers, and families also carry a degree of knowledge of the symptoms and potential outcomes.

Idioms of distress

People use certain terms and words to express what they are feeling, and these idioms of distress vary across cultures and in different settings. The main characteristics of idioms of distress are shown in Box 2.4.

Sensations of 'butterflies in my stomach' and 'my heart is sinking' reflect similar experiences but carry very different emphasis and cannot be easily translated to other languages. It has been argued that individuals who use somatic symptoms rather than psychological ways of expressing distress are psychologically inferior and less sophisticated (Leff, 1994). A problem with such an observation is that it ignores the models of illness used by different individuals. If individuals hold a model that clearly interlinks mind and body closely and they feel that the body affects the mind and the mind affects the body, then it is likely that they will feel and report that mental distress

> ## Box 2.4 Idioms of distress
>
> 1. The ways in which cultures express, experience, and cope with feelings of distress, whether they use emotional or psychological or physical or metaphorical terms.
> 2. These are in keeping with cultural beliefs and traditions, and widely shared within the culture.
> 3. They do not necessarily match diagnostic criteria or diagnoses.

is affecting their body and they may well present with physical symptoms. Similarly, it is likely that use of metaphors reflects a different level of sophistication. Among Punjabi women, for example, the expression that 'my heart is sinking' reflects distress in the same way as some people saying 'I feel gutted'. Like many cultures they also see the medication as having hot or cold properties, needing advice on when and how to take the pills. Often in India, patients will want to know whether they should take their medication with hot drinks or cold drinks and what dietary taboos they should follow. When individuals have these notions of being hot or cold in their body they will form better alliances with physicians who understand these explanations and idioms of distress as well as the underlying psychiatric disorders completely. This mind–body dualism may well have contributed to stigma against mental illness, the mentally ill, and the psychiatric services. Cartesian mind–body dualism has been called Descartes' error by Damasio (1994), but elsewhere we have described it as Descartes' dogma, indicating that perhaps one of the unintended consequences of this dichotomy has led to a rigidity of division between mind and body in some cultures, leading to a sense of isolation across specialities (Ventriglio and Bhugra, 2015). Its ongoing impact on psychiatric services in many parts of the world has meant that psychiatric services and physical health services are often separate, and there is limited contact between them, leading to further alienation of people with mental illness. Idioms of distress carry strong symbolic and cultural meanings and yet may be influenced by the social, economic, and educational status of the individual—and these may change.

The patient–clinician dyad interacts at multiple complex levels, which are illustrated in Figure 2.2.

Once individuals recognize what they think is an odd experience they may ask others around them to see if the experience is unique to them or is being shared. Depending upon a large number of factors, they may decide

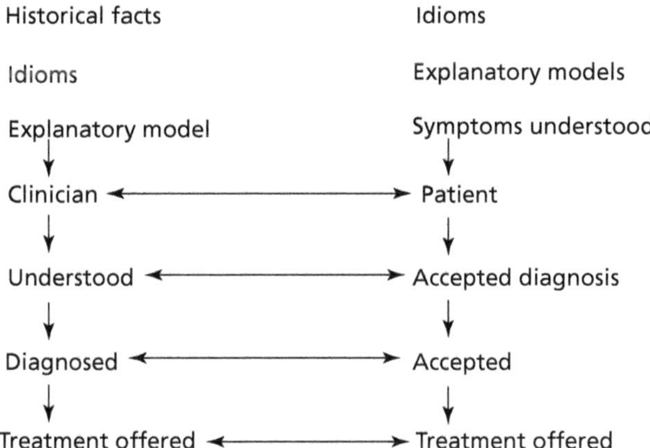

Figure 2.2 Patient–clinician dyad: multiple levels.

this is something serious, especially if it remains untreated. They may give it a name and ask within their social circle as to what should be done. They will then in most cases seek help from personal, social, or folk sector. If the experiences continue to persist and do not get better, depending upon accessibility and resources they may approach the professional sector. The pathway into care therefore becomes significant in therapeutic engagement. This is illustrated in Figure 2.3.

Cultures affect both the causation and the presentation of illnesses, as indicated in Table 2.1. Cultures can directly cause an illness and can certainly help to perpetuate experiences and symptoms. Culture can precipitate symptoms and elaborate how these are presented. It is possible that some syndromes are more strongly affected by cultures than others. Furthermore, the traditional views of culture-bound syndromes has begun to change.

Culture of the patient

It is obvious that the culture of patients will influence the way they think about their illness, how they seek help, and how they identify their potential sources of help. Their cultural values will dictate their therapeutic encounter and expectations of the clinician; they will also affect the way that patients feel motivated while seeking help and whether they stick with treatment or not.

It must be emphasized again that, no matter where they go, every patient carries his or her own culture, cultural values, and cultural expectations.

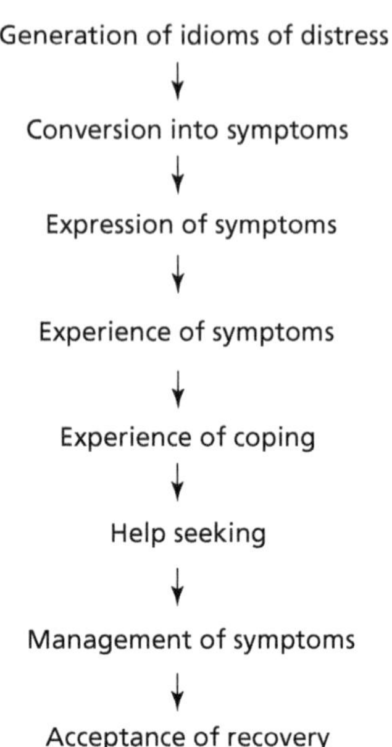

Figure 2.3 Development of pathway into care.

Table 2.1 Culture and mental illness: characterization and examples

Characterization of culture	Effect of culture	Example of illness influenced by culture
Pathogenic	Culture directly causes symptoms	Culture-bound syndromes
Pathoselective	Affects people in specific ways	Varying symptom content
Pathoplastic	Modifies symptoms	Somatization
Pathoelaborating	Elaborates symptoms	Conversion disorders
Pathofacilitative	Facilitates symptoms	Alcohol misuse; suicidal behaviour
Pathoreactive	Modifies beliefs	Conversion disorders

These values are not static and will be influenced by age, social, economic, and educational status, and past experiences with the healthcare system. The perceptions of the illness and therapeutic encounter will all be affected by these factors. Microidentities may also contribute to a sense of alienation when individuals may choose to hide some part of their identities. For example, many cultures hold very homophobic views, so those who experience same sex attraction may actively choose to hide this from clinicians. Hiding their religious values may be another example of managing their microidentity if they feel that health professionals may not be very sympathetic.

Culture of the clinician

Not only the clinician's ethnicity and culture but also their professional culture will play a role in shaping how and where the first therapeutic encounter takes place. These factors will also affect long-term therapeutic alliance and adherence. Clinicians are likely to be influenced by their own unconscious biases and prejudices. These prejudices may apply to religion, gender, sexual orientation, race, or ethnicity. In a similar vein, clinicians may also choose to hide their microidentities from their patients, thus affecting the clinical interactions.

The culture of the institutions where clinicians train and where they work add another dimension to the therapeutic encounter. Clinicians may want to be in control, and patients from some cultures may wish the doctor to take charge, whereas others may wish an equal dialogue.

Culture of the team

Most psychiatric practice and delivery of mental health care occurs in teams. Each team member, whether social worker, psychologist, psychiatric nurse, or occupational therapist, will bring their own macrocultures and microcultures into the team, which may increase tensions. Patients from some cultures may well refuse to deal with other team members, but may wish to see only the doctor or the team leader. Team members may also have different levels of training and experience, thus making the interaction complex. The doctor's relationships with team members will influence team functioning and team culture. Gender of team members may help some patients. Patients, according to their cultures, may find it difficult or easy to talk to some team members.

The hierarchy within the team may confuse the patients and their families and carers. They may align with team members from their own or similar cultures or may well choose to alienate themselves from their own cultures. There may also be subtle currents of different cultures associated with specialities and training within the team. Under these circumstances, the clinician or the doctor may take on a leadership role to deliver the best possible services. Doctors may want to be in charge and may be very individualistic, thus there may be tensions within the team, which may be sensed by the patient and may well affect therapeutic engagement. Patients who come from hierarchical societies may well find it easy to work with a hierarchical team as long as roles of individual members are clear to them. Gender-based hierarchies in teams may also play a role in addition to specialism-based hierarchies. In cultures where healthcare may be privately funded and require payment, patients and their families may choose doctors at a whim, which will add another dimension to expectations from the doctors and the teams. A patient's commitment to a certain doctor and satisfaction with the treatment being offered will also affect the therapeutic relationship.

Other team members may well include clinical psychologists or educational psychologists in child and young people's teams, nurses, nursing auxiliaries or nursing assistants, social workers, occupational therapists, dietitians, and other members in different types of teams, such as physiotherapists in teams for older adults and those with intellectual disabilities, etc. Each of these disciplines will have its own identity and microcultures that will need to be considered in the context of team working. It is important that, within the team, members are aware of cultural and physical hierarchies and how patients and their families and carers understand these. The role and the status of each speciality will form a part of the culture of the team. Each speciality will have its relationships with other members of the team and with the patient affected by their own cultural values and microidentities. Independent decision-making will need to be taken into account when studying or looking at the culture of the teams. Social workers, for example, may be working with families and with the community, bringing multiple levels of contacts and cultures into the team.

Attitudes to diet, foods, and physical activity, as well as to physiotherapy, will need to be recognized while engaging patients. Religious proscriptions and taboos will play a role in the development of dietary habits. Some patients may use their religious identities and other microidentities to engage with or avoid team members other than doctors. The spatial distances between patients and health professionals who may be assessing them are important.

Culture of the institution

Each institution, whether it is a psychiatric or general hospital or a community mental health centre, will have its own cultures. Team members working in such institutions will have to adapt to the culture although it is entirely possible that at times there may be tensions between the institutional culture, team culture, and individual cultures. Microidentities and microcultures may thus inject a further degree of tension. Even if individuals do not wish to, they may have to learn about the organization's cultures and work with and within them.

Patient–clinician commitment

Health systems and healthcare structures will influence help-seeking. In many settings, especially in private care or where patients have a choice, they may choose to take their custom elsewhere fairly rapidly if they do not get quick relief. In addition, transference and countertransference related to respective cultural values will affect long-term therapeutic engagement and psychotherapy. Patients may rely on folk, social, or personal sectors prior to seeking help from professionals. Some cultures may find it difficult to express satisfaction with their clinical services and this may be strongly influenced by previous experiences of healthcare settings. Thus, a multicomplex layered therapeutic encounter starts to emerge. Clinicians and patients need to match their expectations of each other to work towards a successful therapeutic encounter.

Confidentiality

Different cultures also respond differently to issues related to privacy and confidentiality. Notions of confidentiality and privacy in healthcare systems in Western Europe and the USA are very different from those seen in many parts of Asia. In different cultures, there are varying expectations of escort or chaperone during physical examinations. In some cultures, patients and their families expect (without specifying) to be seen together, which may raise ethical issues (Tseng and Streltzer, 2008).

In a similar vein, in some clinical settings, patients and their immediate and extended families will expect to be involved in therapeutic decisions and therefore Western notions of patient confidentiality may not apply. Parents may wish to know all about their children's illnesses and, if the clinician fails to respect these variations, they may find that therapeutic encounters fail, as patients may not engage properly. Doctors must work in the context of local legal constraints and rules about confidentiality. In many cultures, for example, patients are given their medication in the food without specific consent, and health professionals must never collude with such practices.

Conclusions

The clinician–patient interaction is very strongly influenced by a number of macrocultures and microcultures. The first therapeutic interaction between the clinician and the individual who is distressed is of paramount importance because this is when some of the cultural factors need to be explored and discussed. The success of the encounter depends upon the actual purpose of the interaction and whether it takes place in an emergency room, outpatient department, inpatient unit, prison, or at home. The culture of the patient, culture of the clinician, and that of the team will play a significant role in initial therapeutic alliance. Within such institutional and team cultures, individuals may reflect on their microidentities. The challenge for clinicians is that cultures are also influenced by the socioeconomic and educational status of the individual with distress, and that cultural values and norms affect explanatory models that individuals may use. Patients and their families may utilize idioms of distress that have to be understood by the clinician. Specific issues of privacy and confidentiality must also be taken on board as these are also very strongly influenced by cultures.

References

Damasio AD (1994). *Descartes' Error*. New York: Avon Books.

Eisenberg L (1977). Disease and illness: distinctions between professional and popular ideas of sickness. *Cult Med Psychiatry*, **1**, 9–23.

Kleinman A (1980). *Patients and their Healers in the Context of their Cultures*. Berkley, CA: University of California Press.

Leff J (1994). *Psychiatry around the Globe*. London: Gaskell.

Lloyd K, Jacob KS, Patel V, StLouis L, Bhugra D, Mann A (1998). The development of the Short Explanatory Model Interview (SEMI) and its use among primary care attenders with common mental disorders. *Psychol Med*, **28**, 1231–1237.

Pike KL (1967). Etic and emic standpoints for the description of behaviour. In: *Language in Relation to a Unified Theory of the Structures of Human Behaviour*, 2nd edn. The Hague, Netherlands: Mouton and Co., pp 37–72.

Shields L, Chauhan A, Bakre R et al. (2016). How can mental health and faith based practitioners work together? A case study of collaborative mental health in Gujarat, India. *Transcult Psychiatry*, **53**, 368–391.

Tseng W-S, Streltzer J (2008). *Cultural Competence in Health Care: A guide for professionals*. New York: Springer.

Ventriglio A, Bhugra D (2015). Descartes' dogma and damage to Western psychiatry. *Epidemiol Psychiatr Sci*, **24**(5), 368–370.

Weiss MG (1997). Explanatory Model Interview Catalogue (EMIC): framework for comparative study of illness. *Transcult Psychiatry*, **34**, 235–268.

Weiss MG (2018). Explanatory models in psychiatry. In D Bhugra, K Bhui (eds). *Textbook of Cultural Psychiatry*, 2nd edn. Cambridge: Cambridge University Press, pp. 143–157.

Chapter 3

Mental state assessment: Basic principles

Introduction

Mental state assessment (or examination) is at the heart of clinical diagnosis in psychiatry, but is equally critical for developing therapeutic interventions and alliances. Although some of the basic principles of standard mental state assessment remain true, some additional factors need to be remembered when assessing individuals from other cultures. Every attempt must be made not to rush the assessment if the individual being assessed carries a different set of cultural values compared with those of the assessor. The clinician should take time in understanding the cultural context of the individual. Therefore, clinical assessment may continue over several sessions. It is worth investing in an attempt to understand the presenting individual and their carers' idioms of distress, their emotional and clinical needs, and in building up confidence in the therapeutic relationship. Even if the clinician and the patient come from the same culture, a clear period of assessment may be required rather than simply rushing into diagnosis and management. If the language of the clinician and the patient differs, then careful steps must be taken to ensure that there is a clear understanding on both sides of what is being communicated.

Place of assessment

The place of assessment depends upon the purpose of assessment. If an individual is being assessed for involuntary admission to hospital, the needs and assessment will be different from when the assessment is in the outpatient department. Similarly, if an individual has been taken by the police to a holding cell or to prison, then the site and actual process of assessment will vary. The state of assessment at home will differ from that conducted in a healthcare facility. If the individual is being assessed for compulsory detention and the assessment is in a busy or noisy police station or accident and emergency department, the clinician must make allowance for this.

If the individual is seen at home, then cultural environment and presence or absence of cultural artefacts may become important in highlighting the individual's cultural background, and also depth and adherence to cultural and religious values.

Care must be taken to avoid rapid closure of questioning or following medical models too closely, ignoring social and psychological aspects of distress. Privacy and issues related to confidentiality are essential, along with a clear understanding of the actual purpose of the assessment.

Purpose of assessment

A number of factors will dictate the purpose of assessment. One of the important initial steps is how the contact has been initiated, who did this, and for what purpose. The individual showing emotional distress or their family members may well initiate referral, or one of the medical or social agencies may do this. The assessment may be for outpatient or inpatient treatment or for psychotherapy. Therefore, the interaction may well play out in different ways. Involving other carers or family members in sharing information or gathering background information and confirming the clinical needs of the individual can be an important first step and, again, linguistic and cultural differences need to be recognized.

Similarly, depending upon the purpose of the assessment the clinician must put adequate preparations into place. If the individual is being assessed for psychotherapy then, depending upon the type of therapy being considered and offered, adequate and ample background information must be taken into account. If the assessment is for the purposes of a court report, then different cultural aspects and factors will need to be taken into account. In some circumstances, family may accompany the individual and carers, and may provide background information and explain cultural norms.

Non-verbal communication

Non-verbal communication is strongly influenced by cultural factors and cultural variations. In psychiatric assessment, non-verbal communication is as important as verbal communication. Expressions may not always carry very well across cultures. The idea of appropriate physical distance and personal space between the clinician and the individual varies across cultures. In many cultures close proximity is welcomed, whereas in others simply being in the same room is seen as intimate enough. In a similar vein, facial expressions and emotional expressions or their absence may indicate

Box 3.1 Non-verbal communication

1. Eye contact
2. Facial expressions
3. Physical distance
4. Gestures
5. Style of speaking
6. Emotional overtones

different underlying emotions. In addition, some physical gestures in some cultures may be seen as aggressive whereas in others these are calming. In some cultures direct eye contact is avoided, whereas in others it is positively encouraged. Some cultures openly express anger, whereas others avoid it as they may feel threatened by expressed anger or confused about lack of reactions or even feel unable to deal with the emotions.

In a small survey Mistry et al. (2009) found that clinicians varied in their approaches when assessing women who were covering their faces. Some clinicians felt that, because they were unable to see the face, they were unable to carry out a full assessment, whereas others felt that, in spite of the covered face, they could carry out the assessment. This variation indicates partly the issue of cultural sensitivity but also competence in dealing with women who cover their faces with a veil. Some cultures will display emotions in strongly physical gestures whereas others are more subdued. Thus, clinicians need to be sure that they are not pathologizing normal cultural behaviours. The style of speech, including use of language along with the emotion, is also influenced by cultures. Depending upon the cultural groups with which clinicians work, they may require specific training about the ways in which these other cultural groups communicate. Clinicians should educate themselves about the normal practice of the particular culture so that no misunderstandings occur.

Some of the aspects of non-verbal communication are listed in Box 3.1.

Verbal communication

The use of verbal tones and accompanying physical gestures will also vary across cultures. These patterns become even more complex if the individual has English as a second or even third language. Thus, accent and actual pronunciation of the words may create confusion. The use of interpreters may

Box 3.2 Verbal communication

1. Account and pronunciation
2. Style of speech
3. Rate and volume of speech
4. Choice and use of words
5. Emotional tone of voice

alleviate some of these problems but this may raise other issues. Various aspects of verbal communication are listed in Box 3.2.

Facial expressions are significant when deciphering information during a dialogue and more so in a clinical consultation. Veils (niqab) worn by Muslim women may pose a clinical dilemma for the psychiatric assessment, especially if clinicians are not aware of their religious significance (Mistry et al., 2009). It is important that, prior to setting up the assessment, clinicians familiarize themselves with the basic rudiments of the patient's culture. Good clinical practice also indicates that suitable sources of information are not only readily available but easily accessible too. However, clarity and agreement are needed from the outset, so that the patient, clinician, and family all understand the reasons, purpose, and potential implications of the assessment. The rate of speech, volume, speed of speech, and the use of slang or patois must be recognized appropriately. For example, in situations where sexual dysfunction is being assessed, it is helpful if clinicians use the same language, words, and terms that patients are familiar with rather than purely clinical terms.

Cultural distance

Owing to differences in social, economic, and educational status, often the patient may show a degree of emotional distance. Even when the clinician and the patient speak the same language there may exist a cultural distance between the two. This distance may be related to microidentities and microcultures but may also be due to a professional distance. Differences in perceived power that the clinician may seem to have can alienate or frighten the patient further. Under these circumstances, the clinician may well benefit from an unstructured period of emotional orientation with patients and their carers so that very specific words expressing emotional distress can be identified. The use of cultural mediators, culture brokers, or cultural liaison workers who can educate the team as well as the community can facilitate a true interaction between the healthcare system and the community to improve delivery of healthcare.

History-taking

Psychopathology can be looked at in a number of ways (from major versus minor psychiatric disorders to definitions of normality and pathology; see Tseng, 1997). Tseng (1997, pp. 7–9) points out that normality can be distinguished from pathology by experts (using diagnosis made on condition based upon universality beyond cultural boundaries); by deviation from the means (especially for personality); by assessing levels of functioning; and, lastly, by social judgement. It is the latter (social judgement) that is very strongly influenced by society, culture, and their norms.

Careful history-taking starts with exploring the onset of distress and its identification, as well as subsequent development of symptoms. Family, developmental, and personal history are essential first steps. Different stages of history may carry different emphasis and different levels of importance across cultures. Confirming these accounts with another member of the family and from other sources is an important aspect of history-taking, but this needs to be carried out bearing confidentiality and patient wishes in mind. To develop therapeutic alliance not only should explanatory models be explored, it is also helpful to understand pathways into care that will support these explanatory models. In the history-taking, dimensions of symptoms should be explored (Moran and Engel, 1969). In addition, personal history, developmental history, social history, past psychiatric history, past medical history, and family history must also be explored in the context of culture.

Specific aspects of psychopathology vary tremendously according to cultural values and cultural expectations. History-taking is strongly influenced by the clinician's interest in the patient and how comfortable patients feel in disclosing their inner world. This may be coloured by their culture, cultural influences, as well as cultural explanations of what they may be experiencing, as well as what they are expecting from the therapeutic encounter. In many cultures, patients may prefer joint decision-making, whereas in others they may like the clinician to make all the decisions.

Using terms that patients (as well as their families and carers) understand is critical. This allows mutual understanding but it behoves clinicians to ensure that patients understand the questions being asked and, equally importantly, that they double check and understand what the patient is saying and explaining. A successful therapeutic alliance depends upon the honesty of the patient in answering questions, which can make the situation clearer. Understanding both verbal and non-verbal communications is essential while making sense of the patient's distress and experience. A sensitive safe approach is required. Even when the patient and the clinician speak the same language, the idioms used may well cause confusion. As psychiatric interviews are strongly influenced by verbal and non-verbal communication, the clinician needs to be sensitive to subtle nuances of interactions. Differences in conversational styles across different cultural groups need to be remembered as these may lead to an increase in misunderstanding.

Adverse life events

Life events occur across all ethnic and cultural groups, but their importance and significance varies. For example, in the initial assessments of life events in a UK sample, Brown and Harris (1978) noted the death of a pet as an important negative life event; however, using the same instrument Ghubash (1992) found that the death of a camel was more relevant in Dubai. Equally, it is worth remembering that life events are contextual and may be dictated by social class as well as cultural factors, including support or when the support is seen as positive. A flexible and sensitive approach is required while eliciting the impact of life events on a patient's experience and onset of psychiatric disorders. Third-party information may be required to confirm the extent of the actual impact. Racial life events can also influence the onset of distress and these must be explored in a sensitive manner (Bhugra and Ayonrinde, 2001; Bhugra et al., 2001). Assessment tools need to be used carefully.

Psychosocial stressors can be acute or ongoing. Therefore, these should be explored in all cases, but for migrants or those from cultural minorities these stressors may be more culture-specific. These stressors may vary in the context of family expectations and difficulties, interpersonal relationships, etc., and may well carry very different meanings. The stressors will have varying impacts on individuals as well as their families, who may well be the support network. Individuals will also use different coping mechanisms, which will be strongly influenced by cultures and cultural values, as well as support which may be available. It is important to explore with the individual in distress their strengths and weaknesses and their support systems, which may function at individual, family, and cultural or community levels. Some of these will form part of the acculturation process while others can be explored through religious and spiritual values, sexual orientation, or employment and educational activities.

World view

The manner in which individuals see the world around them and how they make sense of this is known as the 'world view', and is very strongly moulded by cultural experiences, values, and upbringing along with acculturation, social, economic, and educational status. Groups within which the individual lives, works, and functions also tend to modify an individual's world view. The same experiences can produce different world views, so the clinician must attempt to understand the individual's world view in an objective manner. This will encourage better engagement, but will also allow the clinician to understand the core values the individual is holding.

Process of clinical evaluation

Psychiatric and mental state assessments are a dynamic process and should not be a one-off event. An ongoing relationship, assessment, and therapeutic engagement involve a number of steps. These steps are related to how individuals experiencing them perceive symptoms, and how they and their families and carers see this as abnormal. In addition, it is important to ascertain how cultures define abnormality. Individuals may experience distress and then, in discussion with others or by themselves, may see it as a problem and may choose to present or withhold information from the clinician. The next step is for the clinician: a) to see and assess and agree whether it is a problem; and b) attempt to see whether a clinical diagnosis can be made within a formulation of the problems. Both these steps are dependent upon the clinician's diagnosis and subsequent therapeutic engagement. The clinician's age, experience, training, gender, and microidentities will certainly play a role but, equally importantly, the clinician's style of interviewing, place of interview, purpose of interview, and familiarity with the symptoms will be important facets in engagement.

Language

The first step in the assessment process is to understand the primary language of the patient. If it is not English then a judgement needs to be made as to whether the individual being assessed is sufficiently fluent in English; if not, then how will the assessment be conducted? Even if the individual is fluent in verbal English, subtle nuances in expressions (in understanding and expressing) may cause confusion and misunderstanding. Sometimes patients are able to withhold psychiatric information in the secondary language but cannot do so in their primary language. Clinicians can explore by asking the patient about their preferred language. It must be remembered that sometimes people may choose to speak in English even if it is broken for fear of being taken as backward or ignorant. Clinicians must therefore be cautious in identifying language capabilities before launching into full interview.

Both verbal and non-verbal communication will therefore affect the interpersonal relationship between the individual being assessed and the clinician. Professions also carry a professional (often jargonized) language, which may not explain adequately or may be readily misinterpreted. Thus, it is good clinical practice to ask individuals to say what they have understood in their own language so that both parties are clear as to what is being said and what is understood.

In circumstances in which interpreters are needed, a trained interpreter, especially one who has worked in the field of mental health, should be selected. It is good practice to have the same interpreter work regularly with the team and the individual being assessed. The interpreter needs orientation to the team. Often interpreters need to provide not literal translation/interpretation but interpretation that is conceptual. Tseng (1997, p. 21) suggests that interpreters can be used to provide literal translation for sensitive topics, summary translations for abstract interpretations, and meaning interpretations for areas that need elaboration and explanation in addition to translation. The interpreter's social status and social relationship with the individual will play a role. Furthermore, sometimes interpreters may feel protective towards the individual and their culture so may withhold information. As interpreters need skills, clinicians also must have skills in using interpreters (Kinzie, 1985) and may require training.

Acculturation

Acculturation is the process through which cultures change along with the changes in the individual's world view and cultural behaviours. This applies to both the patient and the clinician. It is worth remembering that the pace at which acculturation occurs may vary between patients and their families. Acculturation is a multidimensional process. Although many instruments have been developed to measure acculturation, we believe that open-ended questioning remains the optimal exploration of an individual's experiences.

Cultural consciousness

As part of cultural competence, clinicians must be aware of their own unconscious bias and be culturally conscious. There are general common principles of being aware of cultural similarities and cultural differences. Jackson

Box 3.3 Development of cultural identity and consciousness

1. No awareness of cultural influences
2. Awareness appears
3. May be some rejection and resistance
4. Identification and naming of their identity
5. As personal consciousness increases, identity redefined or modified
6. As exposure increases, knowledge change perspective influences identity again

(1975) proposed various stages of development of cultural consciousness. These stages are illustrated in Box 3.3. Interestingly, Jackson (1975) argues that each of these stages has an entry, an adoption, and an exit stage. It is apparent that these stages may not be discrete and may overlap with each other. It is also not essential that one stage be overcome completely before embarking on the next stage. It is theoretically possible that stages may not be consequential and may occur out of sequence. Cultural consciousness should be seen as the process of developing awareness of the culture of the patient and of oneself too. It is about developing deeper knowledge about individuals and cultural contexts. The awareness is bringing into consciousness what is going on and what an individual may well be aware of unconsciously anyway. In this context, Paez and Albert (2012) emphasize that culture in this process is a set of shared attitudes, values, beliefs, and behavioural standards and practices, which characterize an institution, organization, or group. Some concerns have been raised that cultures cannot be known about that quickly and that this is a reductionist way of learning (Dean, 2001). Nevertheless, it is important to ensure that the right levels of knowledge are available and shared so that patients can be engaged properly. Cultural consciousness training must include raising awareness of unconscious biases.

Microskills for clinicians

These skills, although universally applicable for good clinical service delivery, have more specific functions in cultural psychiatry and are illustrated in Box 3.4. To be empathic, clinicians must feel that they truly understand what the patient is telling them. Also relevant is the patient's cultural context,

> ## Box 3.4 Microskills for the clinician
>
> 1. Empathy
> 2. Attentive listening
> 3. Following non-verbal cues
> 4. Sensitive to cues
> 5. Body language
> 6. Eye contact
> 7. Evidence of understanding
> 8. Supportive, non-critical

which will determine how they express distress and how they engage with services. Patients and their families may not accept psychiatric services because of suspicion and stigma. Therefore, it is critical that, using their skills, psychiatrists are able to engage with their patients and their families. It is essential that training enables clinicians to develop their microskills as needed. Sensitive listening and understanding combined with the right questioning style helps the clinician to engage with and support the patient and explore the pathology.

Past experience/history

Previous history of illness, help-seeking, and dealing with outcomes will also affect current pathway, therapeutic alliance, and adherence. These experiences can be critical in managing therapeutic engagement and must be explored accordingly. It is entirely possible that, following previous experiences, patients will hold more negative views of the clinician and the institution. Sensitive exploration is critical.

Concluding comments

Mental health assessment of people whose culture the clinician is not familiar with requires additional time and effort. Depending upon the purpose and place of the assessment, variations of emphasis are needed. There are standard aspects of assessment, but more attention is essential in exploring and understanding the cultural context of the individual and of carers and families. It is important that clinicians are aware of how to work with interpreters and what is needed. Training for both the clinicians to work with interpreters and for the interpreters to understand subtle nuances of mental health assessments can be extremely helpful.

References

Bhugra D, Ayonrinde O (2001). Racism, racial life events and mental ill health. *Adv Psychiatr Treat*, 7(5), 343–349.

Bhugra D, Ayonrinde O, Mallett R, Leff J (2001). Measurement of racial life events in schizophrenia: development of a new schedule—a pilot study. *Int J Meth Psychiatr Res*, **10**(3), 140–146.

Brown G, Harris T (1978). *Social Origins of Depression: Study of psychiatric disorders in women*. London: Tavistock.

Dean RG (2001). The myth of cross-cultural competence. *Fam Soc*, **82**, 623–630.

Ghubash R (1992). *Socio-cultural Change and Psychiatric Disorder: An epidemiological study of women in the Emirates of Dubai*. PhD Thesis. University of London.

Jackson B (1975). Black identity development. *J Educ Divers*, **2**, 19–25.

Kinzie D (1985). Cultural aspects of psychiatric treatment with male Chinese? *Am J Soc Psychiatr*, **5**, 47–53.

Mistry H, Bhugra D, Chaleby K, Khan, F Sauer J (2009). Veiled communication: is uncovering necessary for psychiatric assessment? *Transcult Psychiatry*, **46**(4), 642–650.

Moran M, Engel G (1969). *The Clinical Approach to the Patient*. Philadelphia, PS: WB Saunders.

Paez M, Albert LA (2012). Cultural consciousness. In Banks JA (ed.). *Encyclopaedia of Diversity in Education*. DOI: http://dx.doi.org/10.4135/9781452218533.n160. Accessed 04/01/2018.

Tseng W-S (1997). Overview: culture and psychopathology. In: Tseng W-S, Streltzer J (eds). *Culture and Psychopathology*. New York: Brunner/Mazel, pp. 1–27.

Chapter 4

Mental state assessment: Specific conditions

Introduction

Bearing in mind the basic key principles of history-taking, mental state assessment, and investigation, clinicians must take into account specific factors related to different age groups and different psychiatric conditions. For example, in some cases of working with children or older adults, detailed information will have to be gathered from informants rather than the individuals themselves. Contents of delusions and hallucinations are strongly affected by cultural factors. Assessing clinical insight will be difficult if the patient's and clinician's cultures differ. The role of psychiatric investigation, i.e. acquiring information from corroborating sources, is essential. Symptoms of various disorders may well differ across cultures according to social, cultural, economic, and educational factors.

This chapter looks at specific conditions and age-related assessments.

Patients with psychoses

Patients with psychoses, especially if they come from cultures that are different from those of the clinicians and diagnosticians, may be overdiagnosed. However, studies among migrant groups have shown that these groups have a much higher than expected rate even in subsequent generations. These are said to be related to social factors, including a discrepancy in achievement and expectations (Bhugra et al., 1997c, 1999). Interestingly, another hypothesis is based on concepts of healthy cultural paranoia as defined by Newhill (1990). She notes that, to cope with prejudice, oppression, and discrimination, the migrant whose culture varies widely from the new culture may cope by developing healthy paranoid ideas. This, although superficially attractive, does not work easily, as African Caribbean migrants to the UK (who have much closer cultural norms to the majority culture) tend to have much higher rates of psychosis in comparison with South Asians (whose cultures vary much more and are more distinctive). Although studies have shown that the prevalence of paranoid ideation is high in the general population (Bebbington et al., 2013), the conversion to paranoid disorders cannot be taken for granted. Perceived discrimination and prejudice is more likely to contribute to a sense of alienation and resulting paranoid states.

Key aspects of examination of patients with psychoses are noted in Box 4.1. Cultures affect the contents of the symptoms and the coping strategies. A major point in our understanding of these symptoms is whether the abnormality is understandable in the context of the culture. In many cultures, possession states are seen as spiritual experiences or at times seen as normal responses to abnormal stressors. Therefore, these are not considered abnormal or pathological. These states are acknowledged as such and are sometimes revered. Possession states are defined as a local belief that an individual has been entered by an alien spirit or other paranormal force, which then controls the person or at least significantly alters his or her actions (Littlewood, 2004). He goes on to suggest that possession states can be voluntary or can be actively sought. Described as perhaps the most common

Box 4.1 Examination of a patient with psychosis

1. The patient's primary language should be the preferred language of communication and assessment.
2. Diagnosis should not be based on a single symptom.
3. The clinician should understand the cultural context and whether these symptoms are culturally understandable.
4. If in doubt, seek a second opinion from a clinician from the same cultural background.
5. Explore pathways into care.
6. Third-party information is critical.
7. Learn about the patient's cultural values.
8. Explore the experience of psychoses and possible explanations.
9. Take cultural as well as socioeconomic and educational contexts into account.
10. Understand explanatory models.

culture-bound syndrome, possession states may be divided into two aspects. First, the certainty with which individuals believe that they have been possessed, and, second (this may be accompanied) by an altered state of consciousness (Littlewood, 2004). Bhavsar et al. (2016) suggest that dissociation states and possession states must be recognized through individual assessments in the cultural context. These authors argue that suitability of dissociative trance/possession disorder as putatively universal disease constructs (validity, cultural, and otherwise) really depends upon diagnostic criteria of Western concepts of selfhood, and the impact of sociopolitical influences on disease categories.

Thus, whether these experiences are seen as normal variations or pathological, patients and their families may share the experiences or seek medication or therapeutic interventions. If these experiences are seen as spiritual and uplifting, often no help will be sought. Thus, the clinician must be sensitive to these explanations and be careful that they are not seen as denigrating the experiences, as their explanatory models may well be understandable in that context (Table 4.1). The cultural content of symptoms may well change as the cultures change. In the UK, for example, delusions and hallucinations about mustard gas were common in the 1940s and 1950s; this changed to space ships in the following decade, and was followed by symptoms related

Table 4.1 Additional exploration in patients with a psychosis

	Contents	**Explanatory models**
Delusions:	May be seen as spiritual: positive or punitive	Explore cultural explanations
		Explore personal significance, which may be rewarding or punitive
		Explore locus of control, which may be internal or external
Hallucinations:	May be seen as spiritual: positive or punitive	Explore cultural explanations
		Explore personal significance, which may be rewarding or punitive
		Explore locus of control, which may be internal or external

to CIA and KGB activities in the 1970s. Subsequently, the contents have included the impact of social media.

Several studies have shown that rates of psychosis are broadly similar across countries, although the actual contents of the symptoms may vary. Two classical cross-national studies—International Pilot Study of Schizophrenia (IPSS)(World Health Organization, 1973) and Determinants of Outcome of Serious Mental Disorders (DOSMED; Jablensky et al., 1992)—revealed that the commonest symptom across cultures was lack of insight. However, no allowances were made in ascertaining educational and socioeconomic status variations. There is always a tension between quantitative (epidemiological) data and qualitative (personal experiences). Epidemiological data tend to measure differences and similarities in a somewhat crude manner.

Schizophrenia

The core symptoms of schizophrenia (or the first rank symptoms) are common across cultures, although content, course, and outcome will vary. Clinicians must exercise caution when determining the abnormality of experiences. Hebephrenia and catatonia are becoming increasingly uncommon in many cultures. An acute course with a better outcome has been reported in many cultures, and this may reflect higher rates of schizophreniform disorders (Gaw, 2001). Variations in presentation and linguistic style must be remembered as these may lead to diagnostic confusion.

Bipolar disorders

The expression of mood changes, overactivity, impulsivity, etc. will vary across cultures. Mood may be difficult to express and identify, and mood changes may carry different meanings in different cultures. Similarly, overactivity may be mistaken for 'too much energy' or 'being on top of the world'. Sleep and mood variations may carry different meanings. Expressions of depression and variations in the presentation of depression are important.

Delusions

Delusional disorders show different contents, and care must be taken in evaluating religious and cultural contexts within which delusions occur. Some delusions may be culturally influenced beliefs.

Delusions can be seen as part of schizophrenia, schizophreniform disorder, and bipolar disorders. Delusions are defined as basic and compelling subjective conviction and is not susceptible to modification by experience or evidence that contradicts it (i.e. it is incorrigible), and the belief is impossible, incredible, or false (often called bizarre) (World Health Organization, 1992).

These experiences may be seen as pathological, but can be false positives if their cultural context is not understood. The clinician must explore the culture within which the individual, their families, and the delusions are embedded. It is important that cultural context is not misused. Delusions are said to be present in more than 75 conditions in the USA (Gaines, 1995). This huge range indicates that a degree of caution should be urged while understanding the significance of delusions and their contents. If a belief held firmly is seen as abnormal, is culturally unfamiliar to the members of the patient's cultural group, and is accompanied by functional and social impairment as well as culturally inappropriate behaviour, then it is likely to be genuinely illness-related and needs to be seen and treated as such. However, occasionally it is easy to blame it on culture, and the clinician under these circumstances should resist the temptation to classify this as abnormal. It is unlikely that the clinician will have knowledge of all the belief systems that may contribute to the content and variety of delusions. However, it is possible to confirm the cultural context by exploring these with the carers and the families as well as with other members of the culture, including religious and community leaders.

Contents

The contents of delusions will depend upon a number of factors, including age, educational status, and cultural upbringing. The IPSS and DOSMED studies demonstrated that lack of insight was the most consistent symptom. However, asking about insight and its explanations are very strongly influenced by culture. In addition, models of illness, literacy, age, education, social class, and economic status are also likely to play a role in expressing insight. Stompe et al. (1999) reported that Austrian patients showed higher levels of religious delusions and delusions of guilt, whereas Pakistani patient showed higher levels of delusions of poisoning.

The clinician is best placed using emic models to explore distress and its meanings. The term 'emic' is derived from 'phonemic', meaning that it comes from within, or the way of seeing the world from within a culture rather than observing it across cultures; so cultural values become the key in our understanding of the patient's experiences. As delusions are seen in a multiplicity of psychiatric conditions (Gaines, 1995), a careful exploration must be carried out before deciding whether these delusions are pathognomonic of the specific clinical condition. The externalization and bizarre nature of these experiences also needs careful attention and study (Sims, 1995).

Tseng and McDermott (1981) remind us that the contents of delusions and hallucinations are also very strongly influenced by the background and life experiences of patients. Religion plays a major role in the presentation of psychoses, but also colours the contents of hallucinations and delusions. If belief is abnormal and eventually unfamiliar to the members of that culture and is accompanied by functional impairment or culturally inappropriate behaviour, then it is likely to indicate a sign of distress and illness.

Varieties

The World Health Organization (WHO; 1992) suggest that various varieties of delusions include delusions of control, delusions of reference, delusions of misidentification or misinterpretation, delusions of perception, delusional ideas of guilt, persecution, conspiracy, and delusional jealousy. Other types of delusions include religious and paranormal delusions (most prone to cultural influences), delusions of catastrophe, hypochondriacal delusions, delusions of grandiose ability and grandiose identity, delusions of depersonalization concerning appearance, etc.

Hallucinations

Hallucinations are not an uncommon phenomenon. They are reported by the normal population and can occur because of tiredness, lack of sleep, and after bereavement.

Definition

WHO (1992) defines hallucinations as false perceptions and should be differentiated from illusions, which are transpositions or distortions of real perceptions. These false perceptions can occur in any sensory modality.

Hallucinations in any modality may be accompanied by thought insertion, thought disorder, thought broadcast, thought echo, etc. These can be seen as explicable in cultural terms and may not reach pathognomonic levels. Various varieties of hallucinations have been described. These include auditory, visual, somatic, olfactory, dissociative, or a combination of these. Ethnic as well as rural–urban differences have been reported, indicating that environmental and cultural factors may play a role in the development and maintenance of these experiences (Mukherjee et al., 1983).

Contents

Like delusions, the actual contents of hallucinatory experiences are strongly influenced by cultures. Bauer et al. (2011), in a seven-nation study, showed that rates of auditory hallucinations were lower in Austria, that rates of visual hallucinations were lowest in Pakistan, and olfactory and gustatory hallucinations were higher in Poland and Lithuania.

Spirit possession

Only by *understanding* the processes and how they relate to the categories themselves may we usefully elaborate not only the variability observed in these disorders, but also the reasons for these variations. It is important to incorporate social science definitions of spirit possession to clarify the relationship between a number of salient dimensions of these states, including distress, cultural acceptability, instrumentality, and the definitions of disorder. It is worth remembering that both categories, one psychiatric and the other anthropological, refer to the disturbance in agency, a recently reinvigorated philosophical concept. Possession states are a result of an alien or paranormal force entering and controlling the behaviour of an individual.

Bourguignon (1970) reported that, around the globe, spirit possession beliefs were reported from nearly three-quarters of the societies that had been part of the ethnographic atlas of Murdock (1967). Islands in the Insular Pacific area apparently had the highest incidence, with the lowest incidence reported among Native Americans in North America. A large difference was found between the American continent and the Old World. That no attempts since that time have been made to compare rates indicates the conceptual difficulties of this undertaking, and its relative neglect in psychopathological circles. It would be very interesting to explore this further as, due to the impact of globalization and rapid urbanization, many of these symptoms and their significance may have changed four decades later. Furthermore, as Bhavsar et al. (2016) highlight, to undertake such cross-cultural comparison of any concept, but especially those of possession states, their validity, or truth of its reality, must be taken as a 'given'. In other words, to undertake a comparison of the rates of dissociative trance and possession states between cultures, one must accept that there 'really' is something out there called dissociative trance/possession disorder that may submit to comparison. Well-argued critiques of the cultural validity and applicability of dissociative trance/possession (Bourguignon, 1970; Alexander et al., 1997) are counterbalanced by the work of those who have chosen to investigate variation in dissociative trance/possession disorders between cultures, therein taking the cross-cultural validity of the diagnosis as a given. The extent of this latter work is limited owing to the small number of reported cases (During et al., 2011). Wijesinghe et al. (1976), Kua et al. (1986), and Trangkasombat et al. (1995) have investigated these conditions in Asia. Beyond conceptual issues, the relationship between dissociative possession and trance disorders and spirit possession is important in terms of not only understanding but also delivering services, especially outside the West (Eaton et al., 2011). Thus, planning and delivery of services must include not only the recognition of these cultural differences but training and resources.

Possession states are described as probably the most colourful, dramatic, and exotic, but least understood, and have been seen as dissociative states, psychogenic psychoses, or hysterical behaviour (Somasundaram et al., 2008). These authors reported on a series of 30 psychiatric patients with controls and were able to show that education, marital status, age, employment, strength of belief, alterations in personality, past or family psychiatric history, previous exposure to similar phenomena, and help-seeking behaviour play a role. Nearly three-quarters attributed their possession states to divine forces. Observing a possession state also appeared to have influenced possession states. These authors argue that, in some cases, these possession states are being used as coping strategies to deal with trauma and psychological stress. They recommend that clinicians trained in the Western milieu and method must aim to work closely with religious and faith healers who deal with possession states.

The language, behaviour, non-verbal communication, and interpersonal behaviours in some groups, such as African-Caribbeans, are often seen as foreign and alien, leading to misdiagnosis of psychiatric disorder (Jones and Gray, 1986). Thus, the epidemiological data may need to be interpreted carefully. Cultural nuances and factors may require careful consideration (Box 4.2).

Cultural variations

Al-Issa (1977) pointed out that cultures determine whether hallucinations are pathological. The contents of abnormal phenomena and their potential explanations change with changes in culture. Clinical pointers while exploring abnormal experiences are suggested in Box 4.3. Religion often affects the contents of abnormal experiences and the presentation of psychosis. Murphy et al. (1963) were able to demonstrate that, as Hindu and Buddhist religions favour withdrawal as a coping mechanism, patients from these communities tend to have more negative symptoms. Thus, symptoms may have specific purpose in certain cultures and are acceptable responses to stress and trauma.

Depression

Many languages do not have words to describe depression. However, they do have expressions that are commonly used to express and explain sadness,

Box 4.2 Additional exploration of abnormal experience

Hallucinations:	Spiritual, positive experience
Delusions:	Spiritual, positive
	Negative, punitive
Explanations:	At cultural levels
	At religious levels
	At individual levels
	Personal significance of experience
	Understanding explanatory models
	Understanding locus of control
	Understanding idioms of distress

tiredness, poor concentration, etc. Often, metaphors may be used to describe these feelings of depression. In addition, use of somatic metaphors or somatic terms is very common. Physical weakness, such as the use of the term imbalance, may be seen as reflecting depression. 'Nerves' and headaches (*ataque de nervios*) are common among Latin American populations. Being 'heartbroken' is used as a common term among Hopi Amerindians.

Box 4.3 Clinical pointers

1. Good communication and understanding of the primary language is crucial.

2. Diagnosis may be made over a period of time.

3. Delusions and hallucinations are not assigned to a single reference point but are strongly influenced by past experiences, personality, and cultural values.

4. Cultural variations in help-seeking must be taken into account while understanding pathways into care and making diagnoses.

5. Just because an individual comes from one culture does not mean that they will have all characteristics of that culture.

In the Middle East, for example, complaints of tightness in the chest, feeling giddy, feeling faint, abdominal symptoms related to the liver, and general aches and pains are used (Sulaiman et al., 2001). The implied serious nature of the term may well have different implications. The clinical symptoms and the actual experience, as well as dysphoria, carry different meanings across cultures. Other symptoms, such as biological ones, may also vary across cultures. It has been argued that guilt is a Judeo-Christian concept and is seen rarely in some cultures. Even within the same country, sets of symptoms related to depression vary (Bhugra et al., 1997a), as do prevalence rates (Sartorius et al., 1980). In Chinese culture, the term neurasthenia is preferred to depression (Kleinman, 1980).

In the UK, it has been shown that rates of depression among different ethnic groups originating from the same geographical continent vary (Weich et al., 2004). In a study in West London, Bhugra et al. (1997b) found that Punjabi women were able to understand the concept of depression even though there are no words in Punjabi to describe it. These women were also able to identify the causes and life events leading to depression, but they did not see this as a medical problem but only as parts of life's 'ups and downs'. Their help-seeking focused mainly on going to the temples, gurdwaras, or mosques. This approach also confirms perhaps a more naturalistic and non-stigmatizing model, thereby allowing an understanding of the experience, which is culturally appropriate. In traditional cultures, depression may be seen as a consequence of punishment for not carrying out duties towards ancestors, such as ancestor worship.

A WHO collaborative study on depression demonstrated that sadness, joylessness, hopelessness, anxiety, and lack of energy are common across different cultures studied (Sartorius et al., 1980). With increased movement of goods, people, and ideas due to globalization possibly the symptom profile will change and clinicians will need to change the way they look for and assess depression (Box 4.4).

Assessment

Assessment of depression using standard Western diagnostic instruments may lead to overdiagnosis or underdiagnosis of depression. There are problems with such an approach, as Western research tools may not pick up subtle nuances of depression. It may be easier to explore biological symptoms across cultures, although exploring libido and constipation may create further problems.

Bereavement and abnormal grief reaction also vary across cultures, and clinicians need to ensure that no misunderstanding occurs. In Hindu culture, for example, cremation of the dead body has to take place within

Box 4.4 Assessment of depression

1. Explore whether the patient understands the term depression.
2. Explore whether the patient is using metaphors.
3. Explore somatic symptoms and terms.
4. Explore physical symptoms such as sleep, appetite, constipation, and low libido in detail.
5. Explore explanatory models.
6. Explore locus of control.
7. Ascertain the impact on the patient's social and occupational activities.
8. Ascertain pathways into care.
9. Ascertain precipitating, predisposing, and perpetuating factors.
10. Ask the family if things are not clear.

24 hours and ceremonies take place on the fourth and thirteenth days. For the first 11 months, theoretically no joyous celebration should be arranged. At the end of that period, further ceremony is expected to take place. Thus, in theory for 11 months family are supposed to withdraw from any social pleasant activity. Under these circumstances, to identify all these individuals as suffering from abnormal grief reaction is problematic to say the least.

It is important that symptoms not be dismissed simply based on cultural norms. Culturally distinctive experiences must be distinguished from actual psychiatric symptoms. Depression may be covered by comorbid substance misuse (including alcohol) or with suicidal ideation. Social withdrawal as a covariant of depression may create management issues, whereas irritability as part of agitated depression may allow individuals or their families to seek help at an earlier stage. The role of clinical assessment in reaching a diagnosis is significant, but care should be taken in not oversimplifying depression.

Anxiety disorders

Anxiety is a common response to stress. Fear of examinations, public speaking, and other such activities can lead to flight or fright. Anxiety disorders occur across cultures, but physical symptoms may be expressed in more somatic forms. For example, 'my heart is sinking' is a well-recognized expression often used by Punjabi women to express distress. Similarly 'butterflies in my stomach' expresses a form of anxiety. Various forms of anxiety exist but it is worth remembering that in many cultures symptoms of anxiety are expressed predominantly through physical or somatic symptoms, whereas others demonstrate cognitive symptoms. A cultural context of the impact that anxiety may have is helpful in making sense of exaggeration of symptoms and relevant interventions. Anxiety is a universal experience, which refers to somatic, cognitive, behavioural, and emotional features or a mixture thereof.

There is a tremendous overlap between anxiety disorders and other psychiatric conditions, including mood disorders, somatization, psychotic disorders, etc. It is helpful to understand the basic meaning of the term, which is to express apprehension or fear caused by anticipating danger. The two common responses are related to flight or fright. The anticipated danger may be external or internal. Bernstein (1997, p. 52) highlights aetiological models such as castration anxiety or a consequence of physical illness. Anxiety symptoms may be generalized or multisymptom anxiety or related to specific stimuli. Specific folk illnesses or culture-bound syndromes are associated with anxiety. The prevalence of various anxiety disorders varies across cultures, as well as within some cultures owing to ethnic and rural–urban differences. As in depression, people suffering from symptoms of anxiety may choose to deal with these symptoms by using alcohol or other drugs or substances. Box 4.5 illustrates various clinical factors that are related to anxiety.

Box 4.5 Clinical factors in diagnosing anxiety

1. Acknowledge that anxiety is a complex concept with somatic, emotional, behavioural, and cognitive aspects to it.

2. Recognize the role of culture in influencing any of these four facets. Some cultures may use somatic metaphors more frequently than others.

3. Anxiety may overlie mood, drug or substance dependence, and other psychiatric disorders.

4. Anxiety itself may be an idiom of distress or explanatory model.

5. Avoid misdiagnosing or mislabelling normal anxiety responses.

6. Cultural influences on the role of anxiety should be confirmed with informants.

Phobias

Specific phobias may occur in any culture, but the focus may vary according to exposure. The content of phobias depends upon cultural norms, and the explanation of the phobia may be attributed to magic, evil eye, or another external locus of control. The fear in excess of the cultural context should lead to diagnosis only if it is causing significant impairment or distress.

Social phobias

In some cultures, social phobia may indicate a persistent and extensive fear of giving offence to others in a social situation, thereby leading to awkwardness and withdrawal from social situations. Such fears may lead to excessive anxiety and avoiding eye-to-eye contact. It is also likely that prevalence of various phobias will depend upon the potential stimuli.

Anxiety can present as a culture-bound syndrome. It may also be a part of obsessive-compulsive disorder, which may have significant variations across cultures in presentation as well as prevalence. Different rates of prevalence, differential patterns of recognition and presentation, and culturally influenced disorders all play a role in individuals seeking help.

Obsessive-compulsive disorder

Obsessive-compulsive disorder has been shown to be present in different ethnic groups and in different cultures. However, the contents of obsessive thoughts and actual rituals are strongly influenced by cultural factors and values. Okasha et al. (1994) demonstrated that, in Egypt, obsessions and compulsions are strongly affected by Muslim culture and are associated with cleanliness and contamination, whereas the English sample was less concerned with contamination or aggression. Strict rituals may thus be related to religious purity, and inability to perform these may well create internalized or external anxiety and also worries. As Bernstein (1997) goes on to point out, in many cultures fertility and male progeny are seen as essential and an inability to provide these can cause anxiety. In India this obsessional neurosis (Akhtar, 1978) and in Egypt female infertility (Inhorn, 1997) can lead to the performance of rituals, which may be seen as pathological in many other settings.

In cross-cultural comparisons, the rates of obsessive-compulsive disorder have been noted to be between 1% and 2% (Stein, 2002). Obsessions are related to fears of contamination, harm to self, sexual and religious concerns, symmetry or precision concerns, and saving concerns, which may be accompanied by specific compulsions such as washing, cleaning, praying,

> ## Box 4.6 Clinical pointers in diagnosing obsessive- compulsive disorder
>
> 1. Explore obsessive thoughts and compulsions and their personal and cultural significance.
> 2. Explore the religious symbolism, if indicated.
> 3. Try to understand concepts of purity.
> 4. Explore the explanatory models.
> 5. Explore what expectations the individual has from the therapeutic encounter.
> 6. Explore whether they will be amenable to (psycho)therapy or medication.

seeking assurance, arranging or ordering things, or hoarding. It is likely that religious obsessional thoughts may be more common in some cultures than in others. Box 4.6 illustrates some of the clinical pointers. In the community surveys in the UK (Weich et al., 2004), the prevalence of obsessive-compulsive disorders in minority ethnic groups has been shown to vary. This study reported that among Pakistani males the rates of obsessive-compulsive disorder were nearly six times those reported by the white sample. Living within the same society, these cultural variations are worth noting. Belief in superstitions will also be affected by culture, as will recommended remedies and interventions.

Somatoform disorders

Somatization is a trait or behaviour that the individual employs to express distress, but which may be associated with underlying mood, anxiety, psychosis, and other disorders. The role of presenting with physical symptoms as idioms of distress can often be misunderstood and, if not recognized early or properly, may lead to endless physical investigations, causing more stress to the individual. As mentioned earlier, people who somatize their symptoms have been seen as psychologically inferior (Leff, 1994). However, in many cultures the role of the doctor (as a physician) is seen as dealing with physical problems only, hence those with somatic symptoms may seek help from doctors only. Thus, psychological distress or stress may present with physical symptoms. In many cultures, alternative healthcare systems allow a more integrated mind–body approach. Box 4.7 illustrates some of the key

> ## Box 4.7 Assessing somatization
>
> 1. Somatization may be a metaphor or idiom of distress.
> 2. Cultural values affect emphasis on physical or psychological symptoms.
> 3. Somatic symptoms may be mislabelled, misdiagnosed, and overinvestigated.
> 4. Somatization may reflect other underlying psychiatric disorders.
> 5. Collaborating history and information are a must.
> 6. Avoid cultural stereotyping as physical symptoms may have a physical cause.

issues in recognizing somatization. Chaturvedi and Desai (2006) note that somatoform disorders are a disabling group of conditions, occurring with high frequency in both general practice and hospital environments. The interrelationship between physical health and mental health and between physical illness and mental illness must be recognized. Somatoform disorders are primarily disorders with predominant somatic or bodily symptoms (Chaturvedi, 2013). There is no doubt that bodily symptoms may well be driven by focus on bodily function. Such concerns and preoccupation may be similar to hypochondriasis but, on the other hand, such feelings may reflect idioms of distress that are culturally acknowledged and accepted. Conversion and dissociative disorders convey bodily experiences, which make sense to the individual as well as their families and carers. Bodily distress may result from stress that may be experienced with physiological changes, thus setting up a circle. Medically unexplained symptoms are a puzzle and an enigma to both the individual who suffers from them and the clinician. Hypochondriasis is often closely associated with somatization. These disorders, like conversion and dissociative disorders, tend to follow the individual's understanding of their culture's model or illness, and will not necessarily map onto neuroanatomical or pathophysiological pathways or substrates.

Neurasthenia is still used as a diagnosis in many parts of the world but it is not common in the USA or Western Europe even though until about a century ago it was quite a popular diagnostic label. It remains both a popular and an expected diagnosis in many parts of the world. Hence, it is worth remembering that names and labels of psychiatric distress carry with them certain specific meanings.

Conversion and dissociative disorders

Although said to be rare in Western cultures, these disorders are still relatively frequent in many cultures. Hysterical conversion (blindness, aphonia, paralysis, etc.) is seen quite commonly in clinical settings in many countries, and patients may carry these behaviours with them even after migration. Conversion disorders are sudden in onset, suggesting a neurological, genetic, or physical medical condition but without an underlying pathophysiological substrate or explanation. Conversion symptoms are culturally sanctioned but with acculturation these sanctions may change too. These symptoms or idioms of distress can be seen as being approved by the society and the culture. Key factors to be borne in mind for clinical assessment are shown in Box 4.8.

Dissociative disorders are characterized by a loss of integration of functions or facilities that may be normally integrated in consciousness. Thus, a 'lack of integration' may influence memory, sensory modalities, motor functions, cognitive functions, etc. Amnesia, depersonalization, and dissociative identity disorder are three varieties of dissociative disorders. The fact that these disorders are more common among women means that any conceptualization of these disorders has to be seen in the context of gender, gender roles, and gender-role expectations. Like many psychiatric diagnoses, dissociative trance and possession states display cross-cultural variation and variability both in frequency and in attribution—seen as fabricated in some cultures, pathological or socially accepted in others.

Box 4.8 Assessment of conversion and dissociative disorders

1. Ascertain idioms of distress.

2. Explore underlying pathophysiological and neurological substrates.

3. Cultural meanings of conversion and dissociation should be explored.

4. Corroborate patterns from third-party history.

5. Do not overinvestigate.

6. Do not rush into a clinical diagnosis.

Pain

Experiencing pain is a universal phenomenon, but cultures see it in many different ways and may use the symptom as an idiom of distress. Verbal expressions of pain are very strongly influenced by cultures. Culture also affects tolerance and significance of pain. It has been shown that white Americans tolerated more pain than blacks, who tolerated more pain than Asians (Woodrow et al., 1972; Knox et al., 1977). Gender and age also play a role in the tolerance of pain, as do religious values (Lambert et al., 1960). Interestingly, in experimental situations, if one group is told that the comparator group have performed better, then their pain tolerance also changes. There are also obvious differences between acute pain and chronic pain. A Hispanic group, for example, are likely to complain more about pain and more expressively (Bates and Edwards, 1992). They (the Hispanics) were less educated, more likely to be unemployed and on compensation, and complain of back pain when compared with others. This indicates that for some distressing symptoms social and cultural factors may play an important role. Cultural differences related to pain need better understanding. Of course, pain can also be associated with other psychiatric disorders, such as somatic hallucinations. Some cultural groups are more stoic in dealing with pain. These responses are also likely to be associated with social structures and social expectations. In addition, some groups may use an external locus of control as a possible explanation and may therefore find it easier to cope with pain or other related symptoms. Expectation of the actual role of medication and its impact are also culturally influenced. Box 4.9 illustrates some of the key points in assessing pain. The culture of the individual presenting with pain is as important as that of the physician. There are other factors, such as age, gender, and educational and economic status that need to be taken into account while assessing the extent of pain and consequent suffering.

Violence and risk assessment

Cultures affect the genesis as well as the management and acceptance of aggressive behaviours. For assessing risk, it is important that clinicians are aware of cultural norms in non-verbal communication. In some cultures, being face to face is important and may sometimes be seen as aggressive by the clinician, especially if the interpersonal distance is too small. In other cultures, being in the same room is seen as intimate enough and the clinician may misread these signals.

Risk of violence is part of many psychiatric disorders, therefore making the underlying diagnosis is seen as a significant step. Cultures will denote

> ## Box 4.9 Pain and its assessment
>
> 1. There is individual and cultural variation to expression and tolerance of pain.
> 2. Pain may be a function of idioms of distress.
> 3. It is important to understand the context and the importance of symbolism to the individual.
> 4. The possibility of underlying addiction to analgesics must always be remembered.
> 5. Individuals may respond to a clinician's cultural expectations by exaggerating or withholding pain complaints.
> 6. Cultures will influence 'secondary gain'.

the level of violence to be tolerated with legal sanctions and legal framework accordingly. Domestic violence varies across cultures, and many societies still do not have legal structures against gender-based interpersonal domestic violence. There are major gender differences in acceptability of aggression (Barry et al., 1976).

Violence remains a culturally shaped and culturally determined behaviour (Schultz-Ross, 1997). Schultz-Ross (1997) goes on to note that war is probably the clearest reflection of violence. Interestingly, it has been noted that, even among victorious nations after wars, the rates of violent crime increase (Archer and Gartner, 1984). Some countries (such as the USA) have high rates of gun-related violence and crimes. Thus, violence, its tone, its representation, and consequences vary dramatically across cultures.

Domestic violence may be difficult to ascertain as cultural factors may overshadow both acknowledgement and reporting levels. The impact of domestic interpersonal violence is clear and affects the victim in a number of ways. It also affects children as well as the elderly directly and indirectly. The impact on children needs to be explored. It is also significant that, in many cultures, interpersonal violence against women is endemic and is often subtly sanctioned so people may either not talk about it or explain it away. The clinician must explore this in a sensitive manner. The role of gang cultures and violent radicalization among minority groups brings additional pressures on clinicians. The challenge is to be aware of cultural variations. It is important to ensure that culture is not used as a proxy to cover up violent behaviour (Box 4.10). Risk of violence and risk of harm to self

---

Box 4.10 Factors for consideration in violence and risk assessment

1. Violence is multifactorial and all factors need to be explored.
2. Family and developmental factors must be ascertained.
3. Individual and group cultural identities must be assessed.
4. Specific minority groups, gang values, etc. should be determined.
5. Careful mental state assessment must be carried out.
6. Acculturation, culture conflict, and cultural contraction must be explored.
7. The role of gender must be remembered.
8. Assess antecedents of violent behaviour, including personal and development history.

---

or others deserve thorough exploration and assessment. The clinician's own personality, moral values, and knowledge of the other culture may determine therapeutic interaction.

Suicide risk

Rates of suicide, attempted suicide, and attitudes to suicidal behaviour all vary according to cultural values, which also include religious mores. In many countries around the globe, the act of suicide itself is illegal and it is often difficult to get an accurate picture of rates as well as attitudes. In many religions, for example in Islam, suicide is proscribed, which means that sometimes individuals who may harbour suicidal intent are reluctant to express this. The role of gender, age, and social, economic, and educational status, among other social determinants (e.g. economic downturn) needs closer scrutiny. Sometimes mass suicides take place but mostly the act is solitary.

The concepts of self vary across cultures, thus individuals will carry different sets of values. In a similar way deliberate or intentional self-harm may refer to different concepts of self. In sociocentric individuals, the collective self may mean those around the individual in this context, who may be harmed by the individual's act. In some migrant groups, such as South Asian females in the UK, high rates of attempted suicide have been said to be due to culture conflict. The methods used for the suicidal act and attempted

> ## Box 4.11 Assessment of suicide risk
>
> 1. Assess intent, plan, act, location, expectations, etc.
> 2. Undertake thorough mental state assessment to ascertain underlying psychiatric disorder.
> 3. Explore the cultural meaning of suicide for that individual.
> 4. Cultural pathways into care must be explored.
> 5. Explore the culturally sanctioned motives and differentiate from individual isolating motive.
> 6. Take a corroborative history.
> 7. Ensure that culturally acceptable support is available, which may be from outside the family, especially if culture conflict within the family is causing distress.

suicide are often those that are easily accessible. Underlying psychiatric disorders, alcohol and drug abuse, and physical illnesses may precipitate suicidal gestures and acts. While assessing suicidal risk, the clinician must be aware of underlying motives (which may not always be very clear), along with a sense of desolation, isolation, loneliness, abandonment, and cultural milieu, within which these can be experienced or accepted. Specific patterns of cultural suicidal behaviour may occur and the clinician must be prepared to ascertain these. If the act of suicide is illegal or proscribed, it makes the accurate assessment very difficult. Box 4.11 outlines the assessment of suicide risk. Cultural assessment of suicidal ideation and thoughts, acts, and explanations have to be explored and understood in the context of help-seeking as well as interventions.

Personality disorders

The term 'personality disorder' is strongly culturally biased. There are two current operational definitions of personality disorders based on two major diagnostic and classificatory systems. The concept of the person is said to be context-dependent, meaning that the relationship between the person and the society is important (Shweder and Bourne, 1984). The cultural concepts of the person and the human being as a generic social agent and with a psychological self are important. Obviously, sociocentric and egocentric concepts of self differ. Shweder and Bourne (1984) found that Oriya students (from eastern India) in their sample were more behaviour-focused and concrete in comparison with their American counterparts. These may well change as a result of acculturation.

Cultures affect child rearing and development of personality traits. Inherent values and norms embedded in each culture influence development of world view and personal traits and characteristics. Ethnic characters can be seen in three different ways: ideal personality, basic personality, and model personality. Each culture has a view of what is ideal—the mind of a person any individual should be. Through reward and punishment during child rearing and formative years a personality is encouraged to develop. Basic personality reflects basic attitudes towards life formed by the cultural values and norms, and model personality represents the most common personality (Buffenstein, 1997). Ethnic minorities may carry their child rearing patterns into new settings, which may be seen as pathological by the new community.

Young and Bond (1990) demonstrated that Chinese personality focused on social orientation/self-centredness; competence/importance; expressiveness/conservatism; self-centred/impulsiveness; and optimism/neuroticism. This is in marked contrast with personality traits of American students. Different types of personality disorders exist in Western diagnostic and classificatory systems, such as borderline personality, dependent personality disorder, and antisocial personality disorder, which are strongly culturally influenced. Antisocial personality by its definition will depend upon how social is defined. Similarly, avoidant or narcissistic personality disorder will be culturally determined.

Some aspects of assessing a personality and personality disorder are illustrated in Box 4.12. Semi-structured interviews are the best option in reaching a diagnosis of personality disorder. These may need to be used along with corroborative history.

Personality disorder may or may not reflect mental illness. Health-seeking behaviour by individuals with personality disorders will also vary, as, in many cultures, personality disorders are seen as mental illness and may thus be treated involuntarily. It is beyond the scope of this volume to debate which side of the spectrum should personality disorder belong—cultures do have a role to play and clinicians must be aware of cross-cultural variations. Perceptions of the person by the culture are important and it is essential that abnormal traits or behaviour should not be medicalized.

Culture-bound syndromes

Culture-bound syndromes are locality-based patterns of aberrant behaviours considered to be patterns of expression of distress as well as illnesses.

> ## Box 4.12 Assessing personality and its disorders
>
> 1. Consider personality traits and the context within which these developed.
> 2. Explore cultural norms, values, and mores within which the individual grew up, and consider variation in traits.
> 3. Cultural identity and cultural expansion (acculturation) must be explored.
> 4. Assess social, occupational, and personal functioning.
> 5. There should be accurate and comprehensive history-taking
> 6. There should be collateral corroborative history-taking.
> 7. Culture should not be seen as the sole explanation and the clinician must avoid false positive attributions to culture.

For a considerable period, these were seen as exotic and unusual, and are not seen as fitting neatly into Western diagnostic categories.

Yap (1969) described the concepts of culture-bound syndromes and argued that these included psychological process, reactive and severe. He noted that the psychological process is related to mental experience, bringing about an abnormal reaction in a predisposed subject. He suggested that these were forms of psychopathology produced by a system of implicit values, social structure, and shared beliefs (Yap, 1969). These were culture-bound because their patterns are determined in both form and frequency by the cultures. He emphasized that these were neither rare nor exotic. Interestingly, he saw culture-bound syndromes as a variant (or atypical) of existing prototypes of illness and as atypical of paranoia, emotional, or disordered consciousness. Gaw (2001) provides a helpful subclassification of culture-bound syndromes.

Perhaps as a result of globalization there has been a shift towards moving away from culture-bound syndromes (Sumathipala et al., 2004; Ayonrinde and Bhugra, 2015). In the recent *Diagnostic and Statistical Manual of Mental Disorders* (DSM-5; American Psychiatric Association, 2013) the term 'culture-bound syndrome' has been replaced by 'cultural syndromes' (of which there are only nine), 'cultural idioms of distress', and 'cultural explanations or perceived causes'.

Gaw (2001) suggests that consideration should be given to culture-specific criteria. He proposes that a disorder must be a discrete, well-defined syndrome recognized as a specific illness in the culture with which it is primarily associated. He recommends that such a disorder should be expected, recognized, and sanctioned as a response to certain precipitants in the particular culture, and thus a higher incidence of the disorder must exist in those societies. Cultural syndrome should be seen as a cluster of co-occurring relatively invariant symptoms seen in a specific cultural group.

All forms of distress are locally and culturally influenced and the idioms do not fit into neat diagnostic categories. Although Gaw (2001) suggests that certain behaviours, such as 'type A behaviour patterns', petism, obesity, and anorexia nervosa, are Western culture-bound syndromes, it is noteworthy that amok is still seen as a Malaysian illness, while repeated gun attacks on schools and communities in the USA are not seen as such. In a similar way, it has been noted that *dhat* (semen-loss anxiety) existed in early industrial periods in the UK and the USA (Sumathipala et al., 2004; Ayonrinde and Bhugra, 2015) but is seen as a culture-bound syndrome of the exotic Orient (Malhotra and Wig, 1975). The notion of culture-bound syndromes as it stands is outdated. However, cultural context of distress and its understanding and subsequent management should be seen as important. It is helpful to see the idioms as conveying something that is personal and significant to the individual. Box 4.13 describes assessment of culture-bound syndromes. It is important to emphasize that these do not map on to clinical diagnosis and may yet help in understanding qualitative explanations and form substrates for cross-cultural epidemiological work.

Box 4.13 Assessing culture-bound syndromes

1. A mental state assessment supplemented by detailed history should be taken.

2. A corroborative cultural history to explore whether the syndrome exists in that particular culture should be taken.

3. Are the symptoms a variant of other psychiatric disorders?

4. Are the symptoms recognized as abnormal in that culture? Are they given a name?

5. Diagnosis must rely on culture-specific technology as well as ideology.

6. Meaningfulness for the individual must be explored.

Assessing children and adolescents

The normal child rearing patterns are very strongly influenced by cultural norms. Children are often seen as key to the success of community but they are also an instrument for personal protection and promotion. Thus, the ability to accept abnormal behaviours and the age at which individual children and adolescents are seen to have odd behaviours varies too. The basic biological changes reflecting puberty are fairly universal, but the accompanying rites of passage and rituals do vary. In many parts of the world, there are no child psychiatrists or child mental health professionals. Thus, the need for understanding, training, recognizing, and managing child and adolescent mental health issues may well fall upon a number of other professionals.

Cross-cultural epidemiological studies in the field of child psychiatry and especially in preschool children are fraught with difficulties. The general prevalence of psychiatric disorders using a two-stage design is around 20–25%, indicating that a lot of pathology remains unrecognized. These pathologies must be seen in the context of more subtle underlying mechanisms of family networks, social structures and social strictures, and constructs of mental health across rapidly changing cultures in many parts of the world. These cultures in transition are more likely to affect children and adolescents because they are also likely to be exposed to social media. Social and cultural worlds and their norms and values are important in both understanding what children and adolescents are going through and what their needs may be. Contemporary changes in cultures as a result of globalization are linked with a number of factors. These include substance use and addictions, increase in smoking in this age group in many parts of the world, social media, access and instant expectation of responses, gang cultures, changes in traditional family structures, helicopter parents, newer family structures with various step-brothers, step-sisters, and step-parents, etc.

Pubertal and biological changes are accompanied by psychological changes, in which the individual adolescent is trying to develop self-identity and also individuate and gain some freedom. Cultural, along with spiritual, aspects may well raise other issues. Cultures influence acceptance of interventions and tell us which will not be accepted irrespective of their effectiveness. The onset of nearly half of psychiatric disorders in adulthood starts below the age of 15. It is also known that early recognition and early intervention can provide better outcome in the end. Some of the conditions seen in childhood are more prone to underdiagnosis or misdiagnosis. For example, conduct disorders in childhood can be readily misdiagnosed if cultural norms are applied blindly across cultural boundaries. Similarly, separation anxiety disorder may be overdiagnosed

Box 4.14 Assessing children and adolescents

1. Assess mental state with thorough developmental history.

2. Understand cultural norms and nuances in child rearing, which may be very different.

3. Contextual consideration for psychopathology is extremely useful for assessment.

4. Language, its command and cultural factors in the genesis and maintenance of symptoms must be assessed.

5. By virtue of their age, clinicians are likely to belong to a 'different culture' so attempts must be made to explore the psychopathology and the needs accordingly.

6. A knowledge of cultural rules and norms can help to eliminate false positive diagnosis.

if cultures believe in interdependence in the family and the child may be securely attached to one or more family members. Box 4.14 lists the key points in the assessment of children and adolescents in a cross-cultural context.

Assessing older adults

Attitudes towards ageing and the elderly or older adults vary across cultures. Filial piety plays a role in how people see their own role and show respect to the elderly. Ageing is an ongoing developmental process and has implications in biological, social, economic, psychological, and cognitive reigns. The artificial age barriers in many psychiatric services, especially in the West, often produce an ageist attitude. Biological or chronological changes and ageing are inevitable. However, social roles and social functioning change in response to cultural factors and social expectations.

In addition to the usual psychiatric disorders that may also be seen in older adults, there are additional conditions, the most important of which is dementia. As people are living longer, it is inevitable that more people will develop dementia. It is argued that, over the age of 85, one in three older adults will develop dementia. There are, of course, different types of dementias, e.g. vascular dementia, Alzheimer's disease, etc.

Older people may be secondary migrants and thus may have left their support, social, and cultural networks behind; they may feel lonely and isolated in the new culture. Cultural patterns of ethnic minorities may have changed in response to the expectations of the new society. This conflict with the larger society may also be reflected in the individual's family and the usual generation conflict may become even more exaggerated. Life course, esteem, role, and intergenerational factors may reflect/cause stress and create difficulties. There are clear differences in ageing between men and women. Ahmed (1997) suggests that men move from active to passive mastery, whereas women move from passive to active mastery owing to the ageing process. Filial piety, filial responsibility, and dependence affect intergenerational relationships (Fry, 1988). Box 4.15 illustrates assessment in older adults.

Minority status and ageing may act as double jeopardy for vulnerable individuals. This double disadvantage may further increase if the individual belongs to a sexual minority as well. In cases where older adults are primary migrants or have migrated at an older age, stress related to acculturation may well add to stress. Social, economic, and educational factors may play a role in adjustment. The prevalence of different causes of dementia may well vary across cultures. For example, traumatic brain injury or rates of infection may be higher in many traditional societies. Elderly individuals may still be going through developmental stages, especially as their children may be growing up and leaving home, creating 'empty nest syndromes'. In many cultures, it is assumed that family will look after the older individual and therefore they should be left to it. Mental disorders may be difficult to recognize in some cultural groups owing to ascertainment of age, literacy, lack of valid assessment tools, and various other factors.

Box 4.15 Assessing older adults

1. Use culturally appropriate assessment tools and methods, especially language.
2. Take a corroborative history from family and carers.
3. Ascertain acculturative processes in carers and the presenting individual.
4. Seek cultural explanations of ageing, expectations, and filial piety, support systems, roles, etc.
5. Assess support systems within the family and in the community.
6. Assess cultural identity and cultural distance from the individual's own culture and from the larger community.

Communication difficulties, institutional racism, taboo subjects, failure to distinguish between illness in its own right, or that seen as function of old age may all cause problems in completing a proper and thorough assessment and reaching a diagnosis. There are a number of factors that may affect cognitive tests, and these include culture, education, language difficulties, sensory impairment, and unfamiliarity with the purpose and the function of the tests.

Pathways to care will vary depending upon what older individuals and their families see as the problem and also whether they agree on what is wrong. They may see physical problems as part of ageing and may prefer to see their general practitioners rather than going to see a psychiatrist, which may be seen as stigmatizing. Similarly, forgetfulness may be seen as normal ageing rather than the onset of dementia. It is important that clinicians are thoroughly familiar with the culture and the microidentities of the individual and with the assessment tools they are planning to use.

Assessing intellectual disability

Intellectual disability is seen across cultures around the globe. However, simple intelligence quotient (IQ) testing to reach a diagnosis carries problems. It is important to ensure that, when standardized tests are used, they have been validated for the population being studied.

In many parts of the world rather than using intellectual disability or learning disability, the preferred term is mental retardation or even mental handicap. Thus, the clinician must ensure that there is a clear understanding by the family of whichever term is being used. Intellectual disability is a complex label and involves an interaction between biogenetic and psychosocial factors. Even then the disability is often described by a cut-off point or describing a line below which individuals are said to have the disability. It is a spectrum and should not be seen as simply a matter of social distance. Cross-cultural evidence suggests that individuals with intellectual disabilities are recognized around the world, although the ways in which their needs are identified and managed are culturally dictated notions. In many cultures such individuals may be locked up or punished.

Cultural explanations of intellectual disability include an external locus of control (such as being caused by spirits, as a punishment, supernatural events, misfortune, or gift from god) and an internal locus of control (such as pregnancy going wrong because of bad diet, taboo practices, etc.). These explanations will therefore determine where and how people seek help.

Intellectual disability should be defined as significantly reduced ability to understand new or complex interventions or to learn new skills (for

> ## Box 4.16 Special issues in individuals with intellectual disability
>
> 1. Recognize socially constructed meaning of intellectual disability.
> 2. Explore understanding and explanations.
> 3. Explore the needs of individuals and their carers.
> 4. Understand cultural constructs.
> 5. Avoid stereotyping.
> 6. Explore daily living skills, educational needs, and clinical needs.
> 7. Work with the community to understand how intellectual disability is seen and what is acceptable.
> 8. Cultural communication, including relevant written information, should be made available in appropriate languages.

impaired intelligence, the IQ usually is designated as below 70) and a reduced ability to cope independently (thus showing impaired social functioning). These should be evident before adulthood and have a long-lasting impact on development. There remain methodological problems in the use of IQ tests as their validation may vary. Often, cultural differences get exaggerated and socioeconomic differences are conflated. Furthermore, social and gender roles in various cultures and communities are interpreted differently, thereby adding yet another complicating dimension.

Individuals with intellectual disability have been shown to have higher rates of mental and physical illnesses. Thus, in any assessment careful thought should be given to coexisting comorbidities. Special issues that arise in the assessment of intellectual disability are listed in Box 4.16. Corroborative history and close observation of behaviours are helpful first steps in assessment. It is important to recognize that in many cultures consanguineous marriages are preferred and this may contribute to increased rates of intellectual disability. This practice should not be seen critically but explored gently and carefully during history-taking and in assessment. Sometimes parents may seek genetic advice, which should be given objectively based on evidence rather than a personal or religious attitude of the clinician.

Addictions

Addiction to substances or to activities is prevalent around the globe, although the actual rates may well vary. However, often cultures allow for some substances (such as alcohol and tobacco) to be legally and widely available, whereas other substances of addiction (such as cocaine, cannabis etc.) are controlled in many countries. Portugal and Uruguay have decriminalized many drugs and it will be interesting to see how this affects the rates of addiction and help-seeking. In many states in the USA cannabis is readily available on prescription, raising interesting issues about its long-term impact.

Cultures may express tolerance to some types of addiction for a number of reasons. The commonest perhaps is that substances can be used to raise consciousness or as part of religious ceremonies. Cultural variations are seen as part of the overall attitudes to drug use but also in patterns of use and accessibility of certain drugs and substances. Furthermore, pharmacokinetics and pharmacodynamics vary across cultures and different ethnic groups, raising a fundamental question about the impact and prevalence of substance use disorders.

Rates of alcohol consumption and alcohol dependence vary across countries. In many countries children and adolescents are introduced to alcohol carefully, whereas in others the general pattern of usage is binge drinking. Of course, genetic differences make certain individuals in certain communities more sensitive to alcohol intake, thus creating more problems in side effects and consequences thereof. The assessment of addictions is outlined in Box 4.17.

Cannabis is probably the drug of choice for a considerable proportion of the world population, and has been associated with higher levels of psychoses in vulnerable individuals. It has been recognized as the gateway drug— often the first illicit substance people experiment with (Gaw, 2001). In many parts of the world, cannabis is now being legalized and its sale officially controlled.

Opioid dependence also varies across cultures, depending upon availability and access for both prescription and non-prescription opioids. Other drug dependence widely studied includes that of hallucinogenic substances and phencyclidine. It is evident that there are some main substances of use and misuse in each culture. These substances sometimes carry specific meaning and symbolic value for the community. From a psychiatric perspective, both misuse and comorbidity with other psychiatric disorders are important features. The interactions between culture, substance of misuse, and psychiatric disorders are complex and the clinician must recognize these.

Sometimes substances move with the individuals from that culture. For example, the use of *khat* has moved with Somali migration, or the use of the water pipe with migration of people from the Middle East, and new cultures

Box 4.17 Assessing addictions

1. Take detailed clinical and corroborative histories.
2. Ask the individual for details of his or her last experience, its consequences, and subsequent recovery.
3. Confirm cultural factors and importance, especially religious rituals or taboos; understand cultural acceptance.
4. Explore the first time that they tried the substance and how their experience has changed over time.
5. Explore additional behaviours when under the influence, e.g. sexual encounters.
6. Is there a preoccupation with the substance?
7. Is there increased tolerance?
8. Explore drug use behaviour.
9. Is the individual acting against their own interest?
10. Is the individual self-medicating or taking prescriptions?
11. Does the individual suffer blackouts?
12. Explore the psychosocial consequences, e.g. missing work, problems with the law and with relationships.

may find it difficult to deal with these. Cultures may see substance use as a problem only if it leads to loss of control. Religious values and practice may also affect use and misuse of substances.

It is worth recalling that, often, a proper history will be obtained only after more than one interview as individuals may feel shy and stigmatized. Substance use disorders can occur independent of quantity used and frequency of use.

Assessing gender and gender roles

Epidemiological data have shown consistently across cultures that the rates of some psychiatric disorders are higher in women and it is also much more likely that women are carers for those who develop psychiatric disorders in their families. In many cultures, especially those described as masculine cultures by Hofstede (1980/2001), women are marginalized and do not receive the same levels of attention in terms of social status and treatment for psychiatric disorders. In addition, they are subject to interpersonal domestic violence, sexual abuse and harassment, unequal treatment, and socioeconomic inequalities as part of daily living. Thus, these social determinants contribute further to their ill-health and, indeed, poor outcomes. In all cultures, women are often expected to play certain roles, and these gender role expectations and any variations in performance of these roles may create further tension and conflict for women. In clinical settings, sometimes women may prefer to see female clinicians, especially if they feel that their past experiences with men have been traumatic. Increasingly, there appears to be pressure to create non-binary categories on both gender and sexual orientation.

Female migrants, if confined to their households or communities, may have problems in developing linguistic abilities and skills, and may not feel comfortable with new languages. Racial, ethnic, and cultural differences affect women too in help-seeking and child rearing. Women are also carriers and transmitters of cultures and traditions, hence their role is critical. Definitions of sex and gender and variation need to be understood clearly.

In addition, disorders related to reproductive cycles and ability or viability to bear children may also potentially cause difficulties. For migrant women, assessment of migration, although similar to that noted in men, may carry additional factors and stress. These are listed in Box 4.18.

It is important that the clinician moves away from standardized stereotypes of women as sufferers of abuse or carers, but sees the actual role they play and discrepancy in role playing and the pressures they experience in the context of family and cultural values surrounded by larger society and social norms. Cultural identity and microidentities of women need to be explored and understood carefully and sensitively. Both positive and negative attributes related to female gender stereotyping need to be recognized by clinicians. The meanings attributed to female gender and identity of women are complex and bring historical, social, cultural, and economic factors into play. In many cultures (such as in India and in China), women 'belong to their father, then husband and sons' without individual independence or power. These attitudes are still embedded in the family dynamics without being entirely explicit in spite of the fact that these cultures are in transition.

Clinicians need to be sensitive and explore culturally what is needed for performing the gender roles (Box 4.19).

It is of critical importance that individuals presenting to clinicians are able to express and deal with their concerns, whether gender has caused the presenting problem or has affected help-seeking, or whether they are faced with gender stereotypes. Clinicians must be sensitive when exploring history of sexual abuse, domestic violence, suicidal ideation, or sexual orientation.

Box 4.18 Assessing gender and migration

1. Is the individual a primary migrant or secondary migrant?
2. Was there a period of pre-migration: preparation, family, education, economic status, political issues?
3. Ascertain the reasons for migration.
4. What was the passage for migration?
5. Was there cultural bereavement and loss of relatives, friends, material loss, loss of cultural milieu?
6. Was there trauma: abuse, rape, was the individual trafficked?
7. Ask about occupation, past and current. Is there a discrepancy in achievement and aspiration?
8. What are the current levels of support?
9. What are the current levels of adjustment—language, food, dress?
10. Are there alternative idioms of distress and models of illness?
11. Understand the acculturations.
12. How is the individual adjusting to the new culture?
13. Are there specific issues related to migration?
14. What is the relationship between current problems and the migration?

Cultures may see it as vital that a woman gets married and bears children, and any variation to this role may be seen as rebellion, especially in masculine cultures.

Specific cultural issues like female genital mutilation or rehymenization bring with them challenging notions that clinicians must be aware of (legally and culturally); they must be able to deal with these issues in an empathic and sensitive manner. The role of religion and spiritual values must be explored suitably when required.

Perinatal and postnatal periods have their own rites and rituals in many cultures. It is important that diet during the postnatal period is explored, as many traditional remedies and spices can interact with prescribed medication, causing side effects and problems. It is also important to explore with women what type of social support they require and who provides it. A detailed history of relationships may enable the clinician to understand and explore what is available to the individual. If married, then different stages of

<table>
<tr><td>

Box 4.19 Cultural assessment of women

1. Take a detailed personal and developmental history in the context of culture and personal growth regarding gender role and gender role expectations.

2. Be open to explore sexual abuse, sexual harassment, and interpersonal domestic violence.

3. Take a corroborative history.

4. Explore culture conflict related to gender roles.

5. There may be a need to create and use safe spaces for women.

6. Assess social support, social networks, and support systems.

7. Advocacy and working with a third sector may be required.

8. There may be a need to confirm that individual women are comfortable in seeing the allocated clinician.

9. What is expected of women in your culture? How does it affect the person in front of the clinician?

</td></tr>
</table>

married life bring specific stressors with them, and the role of women may well change further.

LGBTQ

Lesbian, gay, bisexual, transgender, and queer groups are often lumped together, but have different experiences and needs and face specific issues. In large parts of the world, these identities and behaviours are illegal. There is no doubt that cultures and histories play a significant role in the development and maintenance of attitudes towards these groups. Individuals see their gender identity as the internal perception of how they label themselves, whereas gender itself is socially determined.

Bullough (1976) described culture as sex-positive and sex-negative. Sex-positive cultures are those where the sexual act and activity are seen as pleasurable and the main function is to have pleasure. Sex-negative societies, on the other hand, are where sexual activity is seen as purely procreative. Largely, these attitudes reflect and modify attitudes to sexual minorities. There is no doubt that rates of psychiatric disorders are high among sexual minorities and, owing to perceived or real negative attitudes on the part of clinicians, they may not seek help or, even if they do, unless specifically asked, may choose not to disclose their sexual orientation or sexuality.

Clinicians need to feel comfortable about their own sexual identity and should be able to initiate a dialogue about an individual's sexual orientation without appearing to be condescending or disapproving. Sexual orientation and sexual function should form part of the clinical assessment at any given therapeutic encounter. Belonging to a sexual minority means that individuals have to follow certain norms explicit and implicit in that culture, which will have its own mores, values, and nuances. These may cause conflict with the larger culture and the clinician therefore needs to be aware of this. Clinicians may need to be more empathic and explore sexual functioning carefully without judgement. Development and maintenance of sexual identity will need to be assessed sensitively. Some individuals may well be sexually fluid in that they are attracted sexually to the same sex or the opposite sex. The acts may not map on to sexual orientation. Some individuals may see their sexual orientation as exploratory and questioning, meaning that they do not confine themselves to any labels or categories. In some countries, such as India, a third gender is legally acceptable. This applies to individuals who do not identify themselves with traditional gender classifiers. Some of the general key features are illustrated in Box 4.20. The clinician carries a moral and ethical responsibility and must be careful that their personal judgements do not colour clinical interactions. For example, cisgender is an individual whose gender identity, gender expression, and biological sex are all aligned, whereas the term transgender applies to all those who are not cisgender. Some of the definitions are shown in Box 4.21. Assessment of LGBTQ individuals is shown in Box 4.22.

Sexual attraction and ideas of marriage vary across cultures. In sex-positive cultures, it has been hypothesized that rates of paraphilias or fetishism will be higher.

Sexual dysfunction occurs in every culture, but pathways to care vary. In many traditional cultures, individuals or couples seek help from traditional healers or from complementary and alternative medical practitioners. Social, cultural, and religious factors will play a role in both help-seeking and in therapeutic alliance. In many cultures, inability to bear children will direct individuals to gynaecologists and obstetricians rather than psychiatrists.

Spiritual assessment

Organized religion forms part of culture and cultural values for most individuals. The importance of religious faith as well as spirituality is being recognized increasingly and is considered in clinical settings.

> ## Box 4.20 Development and assessment of sexual identity
>
> 1. Find out the age, gender, and reasons for presentation.
> 2. How important is sexual orientation in this?
> 3. Take developmental, family, and personal history of the individual.
> 4. Take a corroborative history and find out about support systems.
> 5. Determine the family and culture's attitudes to sexuality and sexual orientation.
> 6. Is there a discrepancy between the individual and family or society's attitudes?
> 7. Is there dissonance between the individual and their culture?
> 8. What perception of the role and the importance of sexual orientation does the individual have?
> 9. Is there dissonance between their religious and spiritual values and sexuality?
> 10. Ascertain their understanding of gender identity, sexual identity, and cultural identity.

No clinician is expected to be an expert on all religions and their rites, rituals, or subtle nuances and meanings. However, a good clinician will certainly know where to seek advice from regarding the individual's religion and cultural norms. The rituals, dietary taboos, and other factors associated with religion may well play a role in the therapeutic alliance and therapeutic adherence.

Spiritual history should be explored both as part of personal or social history as well as developmental history. It is important to bear in mind that individuals may face culture conflict as a result of their gender, sexual orientation, or spiritual values. Under these circumstances, the clinician needs to explore very gently and carefully issues related to dissonance as a result of individual attitudes and values.

Spiritual beliefs and faith can be assessed while exploring individual and personal importance along with culture conflict (Box 4.23). Religious and spiritual beliefs in clinical settings are often ignored but, for many individuals, these are extremely important. Individuals who present to clinicians may choose to withhold such information, thinking that their spiritual

Box 4.22 Assessment of LGBTQ individuals

1. Check self-identification; stages of coming out (which stage they are at). Do they see their orientation as causing problems?

2. Ascertain sexual attraction, sexual fantasy, sexual behaviour.

3. Assess emotional, social, and cultural preferences of the individual, whether these are same sex, mixed, opposite sex, etc.

4. Assess the degree of comfort they feel with their sexual and cultural identities; are there any disparities?

5. Is there double jeopardy in relation to sexuality and cultural identity?

6. If older, then possible triple jeopardy in sexuality, age, and cultural identity.

7. Is the presentation about sexual identity?

8. Do they feel that clinicians attribute all their problems to their sexual orientation?

> ## Box 4.23 Assessment of spiritual factors
>
> 1. Explore religion in which the individual was born and brought up.
> 2. Explore the degree of religiosity at present.
> 3. Assess how rigidly individuals follow their beliefs, rituals, and taboos, e.g. diet, fasting etc.
> 4. Ascertain if they belong to a kinship or community as part of their religion.
> 5. Are there any perceived or real psychosocial stressors as a result of their religious beliefs?
> 6. Are there any recent changes in faith or a religious conversion?
> 7. How important are their religion, religious values, and spirituality in their daily functioning?
> 8. What expectations do they have from the clinical encounter, especially in relation to religious beliefs and religious values?
> 9. How do they see the role of religion in their distress?
> 10. Consider personal spirituality—levels and actual understanding.

and religious beliefs may be discriminated against, ignored, or laughed at. Clinicians, therefore, must be empathic and sensitive as well as comfortable in engaging individuals whose values may well differ from their own.

When the clinician feels unable to explore these values, either due to a degree of discomfort or not knowing the details of that particular religion, then a referral or consultation with a religious leader (for example, a hospital chaplain) may help. Such an approach also gives a clear message to the individual that the clinician is professional and able to explore these factors, but, equally importantly, that they are taking the individual's concerns seriously and seeking and providing appropriate help. The spiritual history should form part of social, personal, and developmental history, and may well be of particular importance in differentiating religious beliefs and religious delusions. In individuals who may be self-harming or have suicidal intent, such exploration may help them to engage better.

Spiritual and religious factors are often used interchangeably, but they have clearly different meanings and clinicians need to be sensitive to these. By routinely exploring these factors, the clinician may also pick up clues about the individual's social support, personal coping, and social networks, thereby giving an insight into their overall functioning. In many cultures superstitions play an important role as part of daily functioning, and clinicians may need to be aware of their significance and relevance.

References

Ahmed I (1997). Geriatric psychopathology. In W-S Tseng, J Streltzer (eds). *Culture and Psychopathology*. New York: Brunner/Mazel, pp. 223–240.

Akhtar S (1978). Obsessional neurosis, marriage, sex and fertility: some transcultural comparisons. *Int J Soc Psych*, **24**, 164–166.

Alexander PJ, Joseph S, Das A (1997). Limited utility of ICD-10 and DSM-IV classification of dissociative and conversion disorders in India. *Acta Psych Scand*, **95**, 177–182.

Al-Issa I (1977). Social and cultural aspects of hallucinations. *Psychol Bull*, **84**, 510–586.

American Psychiatric Association (2013). *Diagnostic and Statistical Manual of Mental Disorders* (DSM-5). Washington, DC: APA Press.

Archer D, Gartner R (1984). *Violence and Crime in Cross-national Perspectives*. New Haven, CT: Yale University Press.

Ayonrinde O, Bhugra D (2015). Culture bound syndromes. In D Bhugra, G Malhi (eds). *Troublesome Disguises*. Chichester: Wiley Blackwell, pp. 231–251.

Barry H, Josepsson L, Lauer E et al. (1976). Agents and techniques for child rearing. *Ethnology*, **16**, 191–230.

Bates M, Edwards W (1992). Ethnic variations in the chronic pain experience. *Ethn Dis*, **2**, 63–83.

Bauer S, Schanda H, Karakula H et al. (2011). Culture and the prevalence of hallucinations in schizophrenia. *Comp Psych*, **52**, 319–325.

Bebbington PE, McBride O, Steel C, et al. (2013). The structure of paranoia in the general population. *Br J Psych*, 2013, **202**(6), 419–427.

Bernstein D (1997). Anxiety disorders. In W-S Tseng, J Streltzer (eds). *Culture and Psychopathology*. New York: Brunner/Mazel, pp. 46–66.

Bhavsar V, Ventriglio A, Bhugra D (2016). Dissociative trance and spirit possession; challenges for a culture-in-transition. *Psychiatry Clin Neurosci*, **70**, 551–559.

Bhugra D, Gupta K R, Wright B (1997a). Depression in North India—comparison of symptoms and life events with other patient groups. *Int J Psych Clin* Pract, **1**, 83–87.

Bhugra D, Baldwin D, Desai M (1997b). A pilot study of the impact of fact sheets and guided discussion on knowledge and attitudes regarding depression in an ethnic minority sample. *Prim Care Psych*, **3**(3), 135–140.

Bhugra D, Leff J, Mallett R, et al. (1997c) Incidence and outcome of schizophrenia in Whites, African-Caribbeans and Asians in London. *Psychol* Med, **27**(4), 791–798.

Bhugra D, Mallett R, Leff J (1999). Schizophrenia and African-Caribbeans: a conceptual model of aetiology. *Int Rev Psych*, **11**(2), 145–152.

Bourguignon E (1970). Hallucination and trance: an anthropologist's perspective. In W. Keup (ed.). *Origin and Mechanisms of Hallucinations.* Springer, pp. 183–190.

Buffenstein A (1997). Personality disorders. In W-S Tseng, J Streltzer (eds). *Culture and Psychopathology.* New York: Brunner/Mazel, pp. 190–205.

Bullough V (1976). *Sexual Variance in History and Society.* Chicago: University of Chicago Press.

Chaturvedi SK (2013). Many faces of somatoform disorders. *Int Rev Psych*, **25**, 1–4.

Chaturvedi SK, Desai D (2006). What's 'in the body' is actually 'in the mind'. *Int Rev Psych*, **18**, 104.

During EH, Elahi FM, Taieb O, Moro M-R, Baubet T (2011). A critical review of dissociative trance and possession disorders: etiological, diagnostic, therapeutic, and nosological issues. *Can J Psych*, **56**, 235.

Eaton J, McCay L, Semrau M et al (2011). Scale up of services for mental health in low-income and middle-income countries. *Lancet*, **378**, 1592–1603.

Fry CL (1988). Theories of age and culture. In JE Birren, VL Bengston (eds). *Emerging Theories of Ageing.* Berlin: Springer-Verlag, pp. 447–481.

Gaines AD (1995). Culture specific delusions: sense and nonsense in cultural context. *Psychiat Clin North Am*, **18**, 251–301.

Gaw AC (2001). *Cross-cultural Psychiatry.* Washington, DC: APA Press.

Hofstede G (1980/2001). *Culture's Consequences.* Sherman Oaks, CA: Sage.

Inhorn (cited in Bernstein D)(1997). Anxiety disorders. In W-S Tseng, J Streltzer J (eds). *Culture and Psychopathology.* New York: Brunner/Mazel, pp. 46–66.

Jablensky A, Sartorius N, Ernberg G, et al. (1992). Schizophrenia: manifestations, incidence and course in different cultures. A World Health Organization ten-country study. *Psychol Med Monogr Suppl*, **20**, pp. 1–97.

Jones BE, Gray BA (1986). Problems in diagnosing schizophrenia and affective disorders among blacks. *Hosp Comm Psy*, **37**, 61–65.

Killerman S, Bolger M (2015). Gender: a modern guide. *The Guardian*, 29th Dec 2015, g2 p. 19.

Kleinman A (1980). *Patients and Healers in the Context of Culture.* Berkley,CA: University of California Press.

Knox V, Shum K, McLaughlin D (1977). Response to cold pressor pain and to acupuncture analgesia in Oriental and Occidental subjects. *Pain*, **4**, 49–57.

Kua EH, Sim LP, Chee KT (1986). A cross-cultural study of the possession-trance in Singapore. *Aus New Zeal J Psych*, **20**, 361–364.

Lambert WE, Libman E, Pasei EG (1960). The effect of increased salience of a membership group on pain tolerance. *J Personality*, **38**, 350–357.

Leff J (1994). Psychiatry around the Globe. London: Gaskell.

Littlewood R (2004). Possession states. *Psychiatry*, **3**, 8–10.

Malhotra HK, Wig NN (1975). A culture bound neurosis in the Orient. *Arch Sex Behav*, **4**, 519–528.

Mukherjee S, Shukla S, Woodle J, Rosen A, Olarte S (1983). Misdiagnosis of schizophrenia in bipolar patients: a multi-ethnic comparison. *Am J Psych*, **140**(12), 1571–1574.

Murdock GP (1967). Ethnographic atlas: a summary. *Ethnology*, **6**, 109–236.

Murphy HBM, Wiltkower E, Fried J, Ellenberger H (1963). A cross-cultural survey of schizophrenia symptomatology. *Int J Soc Psych*, **9**, 237–249.

Newhill C-R (1990). The role of culture in the development of paranoid symptomatology. *Am J Orthopsych*, **60**, 176–185.

Okasha A, Sadd A, Khalil A, El-Dawla A, Yehia N (1994). Phenomenology of obsessive compulsive disorder: a trans-cultural study. *Comp Psych*, **35**, 191–197.

Sartorius N, Jablensky A, Gulbinat W, Ernberg G (1980). WHO Collaborative Study: assessment of depressive disorders. *Psych Med*, **10**, 743–749.

Schultz-Ross RA (1997). Violent behaviour. In W-S Tseng, J Streltzer J (eds). *Culture and Psychopathology*. New York: Brunner/Mazel, pp. 173–189.

Shweder RA, Bourne E (1984). Does the concept of the person vary cross-culturally? In RA Shweder, RA LeVine (eds). *Culture Theory: Essays on Mind, Self and Emotion*. Cambridge: Cambridge University Press, pp. 158–200.

Sims A (1995). *Symptoms in the Mind*. London: Bailliére Tindall.

Somasundaram D, Thivakaran T, Bhugra D (2008). Possession states in northern Sri Lanka. *Psychpathology*, **41**, 245–253.

Stein D (2002). Obsessive-compulsive disorder. *Lancet*, **360**, 397–405.

Stompe T, Friedman A, Ortwein G et al. (1999). Compassion of delusions among schizophrenics in Austria and in Pakistan. *Psychopathology*, **32**, 225–234.

Sulaiman S, Bhugra D, de Silva P (2001). Perceptions of depression in a community sample in Dubai. *Transcultural Psychiatry*, **38**(2), 201–218.

Sumathipala A, Siribaddana SH, Bhugra D (2004). Culture-bound syndromes: the story of *dhat* syndrome. *Br J Psych*, **184**, 200–209.

Trangkasombat U, Su-umpan U, Churujikul V, Prinksulka K (1995). Epidemic dissociation among school children in southern Thailand. *Dissoc: Prog Dissoc Disord*, **8**, 130–141.

Tseng W-S, McDermott JF (1981). *Culture, Mind and Therapy*. New York: Brunner/Mazel.

Weich S, Nazroo J, Sproston K et al. (2004). *The Common Mental Disorders and Ethnicity in England: The EMPIRIC Study*. London: Stationery Office.

Wijesinghe C, Dissanayake S, Mendis N (1976). Possession trance in a semi-urban community in Sri Lanka. *Aus New Zeal J Psych*, **10**, 135–139.

Woodrow KM, Freidman G, Siegeland A, Collen M (1972). Pain tolerance: differences according to age, sex and race. *Psychosom* Med, **34**, 548–556.

World Health Organization (1973). *Report of the International Pilot Study of Schizophrenia*. Geneva: WHO.

World Health Organization (1992). *Glossary of Schedules for Clinical Assessment in Neuropsychiatry*. Geneva: WHO.

Yap PM (1969). The culture-bound reactive syndromes. In W Caudill, TY Lin (eds). *Mental Health Research in Asia and the Pacific*. Honolulu, HI: East-West Centre Press, pp. 33–53.

Young J, Bond M (1990). Cultural considerations in psychological assessment of Asian-Americans. In JN Butcher (ed.). *Clinical Personality Assessment*. New York: Oxford University Press, p. 112.

Chapter 5

Assessment tools and cultural formulation

Introduction

Inventories, questionnaires, and assessment tools are standardized ways of ascertaining psychopathology and functioning of individuals in a large number of domains. Such approaches have a significant value in providing information, which may help clinicians to understand levels of functioning as well as problems and deficits. It must be recognized that these tools do not and are not meant to replace clinical history-taking and mental state examination but are supplements. Plenty of assessment tools/questionnaires and inventories are available for the purposes of standard assessment. However, these need to be used with a degree of caution as the vast majority of these questionnaires are strongly influenced by cultural factors related to the cultures within which they have been developed. Therefore, these should not be used blindly without ensuring that they are validated for the cultures and groups for which they are to be employed. Various measurement/assessment tools can be used for screening of illnesses, reaching diagnoses, ascertaining levels of morbidity, assessing side effects, monitoring change and progress, and for reports.

To identify the instruments, a first step is to be clear about the validity and reliability of these tools. Blacker and Endicott (2008) suggest that, in psychiatric practice and research, a broad range of constructs are assessed, and that these include diagnoses, signs and symptoms, severity, impairment, family functioning, quality of life, and progress, among others (p. 7). They also note that continuous and categorical measurements are not entirely separable. The reliability of an instrument is related to its consistency and the replicability with which subjects are discriminated from each other—this is largely empirical. Validity, on the other hand, refers to conformity with a gold standard that can stand for truth (p. 8). Reliability is of various types, such as: internal consistency (meaning that there is a level of agreement among the individual components of a measure and that each is measuring the same); test–retest reliability (measure of agreement between evaluations at two points in time); and joint or interrater reliability (meaning that two or more observers will reach the same level of agreement). Validity also has various types, such as: face validity, criterion/predictive or concurrent validity, or construct validity.

While selecting an assessment tool, it is important to be clear about the exact actual purpose of the assessment, i.e. is it to reach a diagnosis, ascertain deficits, or screening for a particular disorder. There will be clear differences between reasons for using tools to assess various aspects. These may vary from clinical or research uses or administrative purposes. To use these assessment tools with minority groups the first question the assessor must ask is whether the tools are culturally valid, i.e. have they been validated in that particular group. It is imperative that the assessor looks at the translation and adoption of the language and conceptual equivalence rather than the literal translation. If the tools are being used in other cultural settings where they were not developed, additional qualitative information may be needed. Kleinman (1988) pointed out that assessors need to be aware of 'category fallacy', which means that instruments developed and validated in one culture can lead to the erroneous use of these categories, assuming they exist when they do not, in another culture. Although there are standard recommendations for translating and back-translating questionnaires, it is important to ensure that conceptual equivalence is taken into account. King and Bhugra (1989) found that, even after careful translation and back-translations of the Eating Attitude Test-21, when used in a north Indian teenager population 29% of their subjects scored over the cut-off point because of conceptual problems. There were some questions that, owing to social and religious reasons, ended up being false positives. Thus, that category 'fallacy' needs to be considered carefully. It is important that, when developing questionnaires, both qualitative and quantitative assessments should be carried out so that information can be supplemented.

Let us illustrate some of these points by using an example. While developing the Dubai Depression Inventory (Sulaiman et al., 2001a, b) we followed a mixture of qualitative and quantitative information. Firstly, we conducted four focus groups (two for men and two for women) in Dubai, in which 40 leaders of the community took part. In each session, the discussion started following the presentation of a case vignette of depression. In the session the participants were asked to outline their own concepts and understanding of depression, what terms they had used or heard being used and what they saw as the factors that caused depression and what its management should be. The terms of expression used were then presented to a second, different, sample of non-health professionals. In the final stage the third group, medical professionals, were asked to choose terms that reflected their clinical experience. Thus, eventually 22 expressions were identified, which were then used to create a questionnaire that was validated against Western inventories that had been previously validated in Dubai. We recognize that such a possibility does not always exist, so a note of caution is required. It is also worth noting that, even within the same culture, not all individuals will respond to inventories developed in their own cultures. The reasons will include educational status, acculturation, and changed perceptions and attitudes due to industrialization and urbanization.

Bhui et al. (2003) emphasize that, to adapt mental health measures across cultures, it is important that, rather than simply relying on the instruments and the clinical condition, their cultural relevancy and validity also need to be considered. There will obviously be many measurements, tools, and instruments that have cross-cultural validity if they have been shown to work across cultures, so the clinician or researcher must use them accordingly. On the other hand, there may be instruments developed in one culture and not validated in other cultures. To complicate matters further, there will be those whose validity has not been tested but which may well have good face validity. Thus, when selecting the right instrument, clinicians and researchers alike need to be aware of these variations. Translations across languages may cause difficulties even if the two languages are close. Furthermore, certain words may not exist in some languages, and so it may be difficult to find equivalence. Ahmer et al. (2007) point out from a systematic review of questionnaires in Urdu that they were able to demonstrate the existence of questionnaires in Urdu but they were not able to demonstrate whether these questionnaires had been through back-translation or had any criterion validity. They recommend that new questionnaires using emic methods may need to be developed. However, to achieve this, considerable human and financial resources are required. Another option is to use the measure from one culture and language and apply these culturally shaped concepts of behaviour and assessment to another without due attention to the cultural limitations; this is called the etic approach. The etic approach (derived from the linguistics term phonetic; see also Chapter 2) has the problem of overmeasuring and misdiagnosing/underdiagnosing/overdiagnosing conditions. Emic (devised from the linguistics concept of phonemic) means arising from within. It is important to remember that, whichever approach is used, the clinician and the researcher need to be aware of advantages and disadvantages as well as the validity and reliability of the questionnaire being used in the same culture. The differences between emic and etic are indicated in Box 5.1.

Box 5.1 Emic and etic types of instruments

Emic: concept developed from within the culture, taking into account cultural norms, values, and nuances. This approach is most likely to pick up pathology.

Etic: concept developed from outside the culture and then utilized on the culture without taking cultural relativism into account.

It is important that the reliability of each instrument is ascertained and compared against a gold standard, whatever that turns out to be. The validity of the instrument should also be ascertained. The domains of cultural validity are noted in Box 5.2.

Instruments that have already been developed and are in existence may require proper translation. These include what has been described as a series of approaches, including the ethnocentric approach (where one culture sees it having a total conceptual overlap over the other culture), the pragmatic approach (which is the commonest, often with a considerable degree of overlap), the emic plus etic approaches (there is some degree of conceptual overlap), and translational (with limited overlap). Cross-culturally applicable questionnaires can be developed using sequential approaches (translating an existing instrument), parallel approaches, or simultaneous approaches (Hutchinson et al., 1997). Knudsen et al. (2000) highlight potential problems and possible solutions in delivering cross-cultural translations.

Box 5.2 Domains of cultural validity

1. Content validity: content must be valid for the culture in which the instrument is translated

2. Semantic validity: words used in both versions should have the same meaning

3. Technical validity: the method of assessment should be the same, e.g. self-assessment should be the same

4. Criterion validity: interpretations of responses to similar items in the source and target languages should be the same

5. Conceptual validity: meaning the same theoretical construct within each culture

Literal translation has a major problem as some words may not exist in the other language and the translation may be literal rather than conceptual.

Clinicians are well advised to make themselves familiar with a number of instruments that will help them to carry out proper and thorough assessments in the context of the particular culture with which they are familiar and in which they work, and it may be better to utilize these instruments only.

Cultural formulation

Cultural competence reflects the clinician's abilities to understand, recognize, and deal with cultural factors that play a role in the expression of distress and subsequent diagnosis and management. Not every clinician will be proficient in every culture, but they should have the skills and ability to recognize some common basic principles and have the competencies to explore cultural similarities and differences. Cultural competency is also about recognizing one's own cultural strengths and weaknesses, including prejudices. It is likely that in many settings patients and clinicians will come from different ethnic and cultural backgrounds, as well as gender and religion, and these may create unrecognized and unconscious biases and tensions on both sides, leading to poor engagement. Thus, clinicians must be aware of their own microidentities and those of the patients. Even within the same broad culture, there will be microcultures, which are likely to affect verbal and non-verbal communication. It must also be recognized and remembered that cultures are never static, but are dynamic, and the changes will affect individuals and their communities. Having proficiency in different languages may reduce the need for interpreters. However, some patients from a culture may prefer to see a clinician from the same background because they feel comforted, whereas others may feel that by being ill they are bringing shame on their culture so would rather see someone not familiar with their culture. When interpreters are used, it is important that they are trained, and clinicians should try to work with the same interpreter if possible so that both can get used to each other and agree a way of working together. There is no doubt that working with interpreters requires a different set of skills, and clinicians and their teams must be aware of specific issues and should be trained in the use of interpreters.

Cultural competence works at different levels. At the heart of the therapeutic interaction is the clinical competence of the clinician, then that of the team, and the overarching competence is that of the organization or the institution within which the clinician is working and where patients are seen. A key part of this clinical competence is cultural competence. Following a systematic review, Bhui et al. (2007) observed that cultural competence includes modifications of clinical practice and organizational performance, thus working at both individual and institutional levels. One model of cultural competence is that of cultural consultation, which shows a change in attitudes and skills of staff. These authors note that knowledge of cultural values, beliefs, and practices are indeed necessary for the clinician, because otherwise the likelihood of underdiagnosis and misdiagnosis increases, which may lead to poorer outcomes and poor therapeutic engagement. There are various methods of learning and being culturally competent; these may be through didactic teaching and lectures, role-play, case discussion, and clinical cases through teaching by patients. It is imperative that organizations too become culturally competent, and this must be embedded in the infrastructure and ethos of any service provider (Bhui et al., 2007). Without such an approach, individual clinical practice can change only so much and may not be sustainable. Culture brokers, culture mediators, and culture ambassadors all have a role to play in liaising with the community on the one hand and with the service providers on the other. Individuals in these roles can educate the patients using the services, their carers and families, and the teams about the cultural groups they are meant to be serving, thereby creating a conduit for dialogue. Organizations, which are seen as culturally competent, also work closely with other organizations as well as traditional healers, faith healers, religious leaders, and other stakeholders.

Cultural formulation is now an integral part of the *Diagnostic and Statistical Manual of Mental Disorders* (DSM-5; American Psychiatric Association, 2013) and relies on what is required within DSM-5 to reach clinical diagnosis. In this chapter, we provide a brief overview of cultural formulation from a DSM-5 perspective and then outline what others need to know. Cultural formulation brings together various aspects of psychopathology, history, and investigations into the context of cultural values and norms so that appropriate therapeutic interventions can then be set in place. There has been a major debate on the concepts of cultural formulation and its utility in psychiatry.

Gaw (2001) provides a helpful introduction to cultural formulation, looking at cultural identity of the individual; cultural explanations of the individual's illness, psychosocial environment, and levels of functioning; cultural elements embedded within the therapeutic encounter between the clinician and the individual with distress; and overall cultural assessment for diagnosis and care.

Cultural formulation is a set of guidelines that clinicians use as a cultural analysis process relating to every clinical encounter (Lewis-Fernandez, 1996; Lewis-Fernandez et al., 2014). Its purpose is to assist and enable the clinician to evaluate systematically and report the impact of individuals' cultural context on how they experience their illness and what sense they make of it. Through an appreciation of the cultural perspective in the process of assessment, the clinician may be better able to understand the context within which the distressed individual is going through their illness experience and what sense they make of it. There is every likelihood that such an approach will allow a better understanding of what is seen and recognized as normal or abnormal. The challenge really is to apply cultural formulation to *all* patients. Often erroneously, the concept of cultural formulation is applied only to those individuals whose cultures differ from that of the clinician or those who are simply from minority cultures.

The outline of cultural formulation in DSM-5 includes a systematic review of a patient's life experience in a number of areas. These areas include: (i) the individual's cultural background; (ii) the role of cultural context in the expression and evaluation of symptoms and dysfunction; and (iii) the effect of these cultural differences on the relationship between the individual and the clinician.

Psychiatric assessment, like all medical assessments, depends upon thorough history-taking with corroborating history, mental state assessment, and investigations, which may include medical, psychological, and social investigations.

Kleinman (1988) recommends associate interview where the individual in distress is encouraged to speak freely and continuously while the interviewer subtly provides direction; the exploration is through the use of open-ended questions. According to Gaw (2001), such an approach allows information to flow naturally from individuals in distress, thus avoiding clinician/interviewer bias, and conveys a clear message to the individual that all this information is relevant to their experience (and significant to the clinician). This also encourages the clinician to be open-minded and explore various issues, including models and symptoms, without asking direct and closed questions. Following the initial recognition and the importance of the presenting complaint, the social and cultural settings must be explored. On occasion, it may be easier to start with an exploration of cultural values and identity, and then narrow down to symptoms and distress. It depends upon the style and personality of the clinician as well as that of the patient. Part of the clinical assessment depends upon the clinician building rapport with the individual in distress. It is always useful to recognize that individuals in distress and their carers and family members may feel stigmatized against and experience prejudice in seeking help, which may delay help-seeking or engagement. The clinician must be aware of their own prejudices and strengths as well as weaknesses.

The cultural identity of the individual will require specific explorations and some of the relevant areas are given in Box 5.3.

Clinicians also need to be aware of the phenomenon of cultural contraction. Cultural contraction is defined as individuals giving up various aspects of their own culture voluntarily or otherwise. Cultural expansion, on the other hand, will include learning about new cultures, adapting to them, and absorbing aspects, which may be easier to understand, assimilate, and may be seen as necessary for being accepted in the new culture. Both of these phenomena are an essential part of the process of acculturation.

Exploration of the experience of migration (which not every individual will have gone through) requires specific sensitivity. Some of the areas to be ascertained in interview are listed in Box 5.4.

Assessment of cultural concepts of distress or explanatory models can enable clinicians to determine the dissonance between their world view and those of the individual who is presenting with distress, along with those of the carers and families who may be looking after the individual. Carabello et al. (2015) provide further details of exploration of the cultural concepts of

Box 5.3 Cultural identity

1. Gender
2. Race
3. Ethnicity
4. Country of origin
5. Culture of origin: how would they describe themselves?
6. Primary language: spoken at home/at work/at leisure?
7. Sexual orientation
8. Marital status: age at which married/arranged marriage?
9. Religious and spiritual beliefs: organized religion? Religious leader from same ethnicity?
10. Educational achievement
11. Level of employment
12. Social/economic status
13. History of migration, if applicable
14. Acculturation
15. Degree of comfort in own culture and in larger society

Box 5.4 Assessing migration and associated experiences

1. When? How old?
2. Alone or in a group?
3. With or without family members?
4. Primary migrant?
5. Secondary migrant?
6. Support structures?
7. Language skills?
8. Employment
9. Financial status
10. Aspirations in areas of education, housing, social status, employment, etc.
11. Achievements in the above areas

distress. They suggest exploring symptoms, precipitators and explanations, severity and level of dysfunction, history of past treatment, and experience of help-seeking.

DSM-5 provides further details of cultural formulation and cultural formulation interviews (CFIs) and supplementary modules. It is important to follow the structures recommended, but a degree of flexibility may well be required within these structures. Lewis-Fernandez et al. (2014) describe the outline for cultural formulation (OCF) and the questions asked in the CFI. Some of these categories are illustrated in Box 5.5. These authors provide a background on the development of the concept of cultural formulation in

Box 5.5 Cultural formulation categories

1. Cultural definition of the problem
2. Cultural perceptions of the cause, context, and support
3. Cultural factors affecting self-coping and past help-seeking
4. Cultural factors affecting current help-seeking
5. Relationship with the patient

DSM-5. They point out that the publication of the OCF in the last edition of the DSM was a milestone for cultural psychiatry, acknowledging culture's relevance to mainstream psychiatry. The OCF was a concise list of cultural topics organized by broad domains for clinicians to consider in the assessment of patients. The key features include cultural identity of individuals, cultural explanations of their illness, cultural factors related to their environment and levels of functioning, various cultural elements of relationship between the clinician and the individual, and overall cultural assessment. Taking these dimensions into account, cultural formulation can be produced. The key elements of the CFI are listed in Box 5.5. Similar areas are to be explored with the informants.

DSM-5 recommends that similar areas be explored with the informant because cultural concepts are important in psychiatric diagnosis for several reasons: to avoid misdiagnosis, to obtain useful clinical information, improve clinical rapport and engagement, and therapeutic efficacy, as well as to clarify cultural epidemiology and research questions (American Psychiatric Association, 2013, pp. 758–759). For the first time DSM suggests that cultural concepts should determine whether they meet the diagnostic criteria for a specified disorder or *other specified or unspecified* diagnosis.

It is important that clinicians use a clear and culturally sensitive approach in using assessment tools as well as history-taking and mental state assessment so that management and therapeutic interventions are clear, appropriate, and useful. Using tools such as the CFI, the clinician can explore basic psychopathology and improve therapeutic alliance. A culturally orientated assessment and interview will certainly contribute to better engagement and help reduce the alienation that is felt by and reported by black and ethnic minority populations in many countries. Such an approach will add to patient satisfaction. The fact that the clinician is interested in exploring the patient's background and cultural models of distress will emphasize that the clinician is committed to understanding the patient as a whole individual, their experiences and understanding, thereby providing an element of equality and equity. Research methods and recruitment may thus be better standardized.

References

Ahmer S, Faruqui RA, Aijaz A (2007). Psychiatric rating scales in Urdu: a systematic review. *BMC Psychiatry*, 7, 59.

American Psychiatric Association (2013). *Diagnostic and Statistical Manual of Mental Disorders*, 5th edn (DSM-5). Washington, DC: APPI.

Bhui K, Mohamud S, Warfa N, Craig TJ, Stansfeld S (2003). Cultural adaptation of mental health measures: improving the quality of clinical practice and research. *Br J Psych*, **183**, 184–186.

Bhui K, Warfa N, Edonyo P, McKenzie K, Bhugra D (2007). Cultural competence in mental health care: a review of model evaluations. *BMC Health Services Research*, **7**, 15.

Blacker D, Endicott J (2008). Psychometric properties: concepts of reliability and validity. In: AJ Rush, M First, and D Blacker (eds). *Handbook of Psychometric Measures*. Washington, DC: APPI, pp. 7–14.

Carabello A, Lee JR, Lim RF (2015). Applying the DSM-5 outline for cultural formulation and the cultural formulations interview. In RF Lim (ed). *Clinical Manual of Cultural Psychiatry*. Washington, DC: APPI, pp. 43–76.

Gaw AC (2001). *Cross-Cultural Psychiatry*. Washington, DC: American Psychiatric Publishing.

Hutchinson A, Bentzen N, Konig-Zahn C (1997). *Cross Cultural Health Outcome Assessment: A User's Guide*, vol. **1**. Ruinen: European Research Group Health Outcomes.

King M, Bhugra D (1989). Eating disorders: lessons from cross-cultural study. *Psychol Med*, **19**, 955–958.

Kleinman A (1988). *Rethinking Psychiatry: From Cultural Category to Personal Experience*. New York: Free Press.

Knudsen H, Vazquez-Barqueio JL, Wlcher B, et al. (2000). Translation and cross-cultural adaption of outcome measurements for schizophrenia Epsilon Study. *Br J Psych*, **177**, 58–514.

Lewis-Fernandez R (1996). Cultural formulation of psychiatric diagnosis. *Cult Med Psych*, **20**, 133–144.

Lewis-Fernandez R, Aggarwal NK, Baarnhielm S, et al. (2014). Culture and psychiatric evaluation: operationalizing cultural formulation for DSM-5. *Psychiatry*, **77**, 130–154.

Sulaiman S, Bhugra D, de Silva P (2001a). Perceptions of depression in a community sample in Dubai. *Transcult Psych*, **38**, 201–218.

Sulaiman S, Bhugra D, de Silva P (2001b). The development of a culturally sensitive symptom checklist for depression in Dubai. *Transcult Psych*, **38**, 219–229.

Chapter 6

Psychopharmacology and culture

Introduction

Medication as part of the therapeutic encounter, whether prescribed or bought over the counter (OTC), plays a major role in managing various types of distress and symptoms that lead to illness. Expectations of what medications are for and what they actually do vary across cultures. Individuals may well have tried medication or some variant of it prior to approaching the formal professional health sector. Help-seeking depends upon a number of factors, including what the explanatory models are and what resources are available and accessible. Most often the first step in help-seeking is within the personal, folk, or social sectors. Depending upon access to the formal healthcare system, availability of healthcare, and type of healthcare systems individuals will seek help from the professional sector. The rules for prescription medicines vary across cultures. In many settings, a lot of prescription-only medicines can be easily bought OTC. In many cultures, individuals may well be simultaneously using complementary and alternative medicines. Thus, a clear understanding of the role of medication, its symbolic significance and meaning to the individual, along with the importance the patient gives to the medication is needed. To complicate matters further regarding medication, for a considerable length of time the development and drug trials of new drugs has been carried out in high-income countries, and thus often very little attention is paid to the cultural and ethnic differences in the use and importance of medication. It is only in the past three decades or so that increasing attention is being paid to cultural, ethnic, and racial differences in the use of medications. The reasons for such variations in the use and responses are many and include pharmacodynamic and pharmacokinetic factors but also various non-biological factors such as diet, smoking leading to interactions with tobacco, complementary and alternative medicine, religious taboos and rituals, and other environmental factors.

General factors

It is helpful to understand some of the basic general factors that affect use and acceptance of medication. These include racial and ethnic variations, which are related to biological, psychological, and cultural factors. We should remind ourselves that individuals belonging to a particular ethnicity or culture share language, religion, values, and world view. They may carry with them taboos, folk memory, etc. that are all shared experiences and influence an individual's ethnic identity. The wide range of features involved in various definitions of ethnicity and sometimes cultures, especially microidentities, reflect various biological and social factors which will affect as well as influence acceptance of certain types of medication and dietary interactions. The role of clinicians and the perceived and real power they hold carries with it cultural values too. There are, of course, problems in epidemiological studies using ethnicity or race as a variable as neither of these terms map neatly on to culture.

There is no doubt that evidence-based medicine is important but, if drug trials and treatment guidelines rely on white majority populations without taking biological and cultural diversity into account, these may have very limited applications to other cultures. Little is known regarding the potential contribution of cultural (racial and ethnic) factors in determining whether a particular medication or treatment regime will be helpful in treating a particular patient with a specific condition (even if the actual symptoms are similar) (Lin, 1996). This has caused neglect in understanding biological diversity and factors influencing metabolism.

Treatment planning is outlined in Box 6.1.

Personality factors

Personality is strongly influenced by child rearing patterns, which in turn are very strongly affected by culture. Similarly, both culture and personality will mould the therapeutic encounter and the expectations that individuals in distress or their carers and families may have in these situations. In many cultures the physician is seen as the ultimate arbiter, and individual patients may allow decisions to be made on their behalf, whereas in other cultures they may want to have equal partnership and equal say in making decisions which affect them. Furthermore, culturally determined personality traits such as interdependence, orthodoxy, etc. (along with physical/biological factors such as height, body mass, weight) will affect drug metabolism, as well as subjective responses, which are all major parts of pharmacodynamics and pharmacokinetics (Lin et al., 1995). It is important that clinicians do

---

Box 6.1 Implementing the treatment plan

1. Convey the diagnosis to the individual and the carers—check that they have understood—use written information as a supplement.

2. Explain the therapeutic intervention—drugs and talking therapies—ensure that they have understood.

3. Ensure that they follow the advantages and disadvantages (i.e. side effects) of drugs or therapies.

4. Assess how these map into individuals' and their families' expectations and explanatory models.

5. Give detailed written information on interactions and avoidance of foods, etc.

6. Offer follow-up discussions with yourself, other trained professionals, or pharmacists.

7. Ensure thorough assessment, choose medication carefully, check serum levels or metabolizer status if possible.

---

not follow Eurocentric or Caucasocentric approaches at both cultural and medicinal levels. Not considering individual factors affects therapeutic engagement as well as outcome.

Environmental factors

Many environmental factors—especially related to culture—can cause changes in the pharmacodynamics and pharmacokinetics of prescribed medication. Some of these are internal cultural factors such as proscription of tobacco use among Sikhs, whereas others may be associated with diet, religious taboos, and ease of access to OTC medication. In countries and cultures where OTC medication is easily available, cheap, and accessible, patients and their families may prefer those than going to the doctor and seeking prescriptions. The access and use of alternative and complementary medicine may well lead to drug interactions if the prescribing physician is not aware of what the patient may be taking. Nicotine, food additives, caffeine, environmental pollution, etc. may well influence both pharmacokinetics and pharmacodynamics (Westermeyer, 1989). These variations are mediated by both genetic and non-genetic factors (Ng et al., 2004). Lin and Smith (2000) suggest that, often, genetic or biological factors may be ignored while instituting drug therapy. Higher levels of stress and lower levels of social support may affect therapeutic dosages and therapeutic levels of medication and these people thus have poorer outcomes. Across generations, environmental factors may induce genetic changes, which will further influence the outcome.

The role that carers and family can play in building up the therapeutic alliance and supporting medication intake cannot be underestimated.

Ng and Bousman (2018) observe that psychiatrists often use a unidimensional view of the patient by applying a categorical approach to prescribing medications (such as diagnostic subtypes, compliance–non-compliance, response–non-response, etc.). Even when clinicians are sensitive to cultural or ethnic factors there appears to be an assumption that all recipients have the same biological factors. It must be recognized that there will be individual variations even within the same cultural or ethnic groups, so specific attention must be paid to individual metabolic function based on age, gender, hepatic and renal function, body weight, etc.

Culture and the placebo effect

The placebo response relates to the use of inert substances that may produce helpful or unhelpful changes. Placebos work as psychological instruments both for the patient and for the clinician. It has been argued that, at times, between 30% and 70% of the therapeutic response obtained with any treatment method may well be due to the placebo phenomenon (Smith et al., 1993), although it is only recently that such phenomena have been studied across cultural groups. Such actions are attributable both to the symbolic interaction, which is the taking and giving of the medication, as well as faith in the prescribing physician and the actual medicine. Both aspects are strongly influenced by cultural factors. The actual impact of placebo is not entirely clear in drug trials but what is clear is that culture influences an individual's response to placebo. Bhugra and Ventriglio (2015) suggest that expectancy of response and expectations embedded in the clinician play a role in the placebo response. Placebos offer psychological and physiological effect of meanings.

In some cultures, individuals prefer liquid medication whereas, in others, injections or capsules are preferable. In some cultures, blue is seen as a calming colour so blue tablets are preferred if the individual feels agitated, whereas in others individuals prefer green or red coloured tablets as these colours have special significance. Caucasian Americans see white capsules as having analgesic properties, whereas African Americans see white capsules as having stimulant properties. Caucasians see black capsules as stimulants, whereas African Americans see these as analgesics (Buckalew and Coffield,

1982). In many cultures, medication is seen to have either hot or cold properties, as do various types of food, so the individuals who require medication will seek clarification on dietary restrictions and dietary interactions. Patients expect that their doctors not only agree with these notions but will also know such interactions and will be able to advise accordingly. If such advice is not forthcoming, patients may not take therapeutic intervention seriously. Clinicians therefore need to be aware of the cultural expectations and the potential explanatory models and the implications and symbols embedded in medication and its effects.

Complementary and alternative medicines

Explanatory models related to the illness will influence where the patients and their families seek help from and whether they follow the advice offered. Many cultural groups may well prefer traditional or non-Western medications. As mentioned earlier, if access to the Western healthcare system is expensive or difficult then the first port of call may well be traditional medicine. Many of these medications from Ayurvedic, Chinese, or Unani systems contain high levels of psychoactive substances that can lead to higher levels of side effects and subsequent rejection of prescribed medication, with patients attributing ill effects to Western medication rather than the interaction. Alternative medications may also contain high levels of zinc, lead, mercury, antimony, and other metals, which may cause further problems. In many cultures, these are seen as herbal medicines which, because they are 'natural', will be seen as having no side effects—the reality is that they may contain psychoactive compounds which will interact with prescribed medications.

Practitioners of alternative medicine may also recommend food restrictions and taboos so that absorption of these medications can be improved. If an allopathic physician is not aware of these restrictions and the active components of medication, the likelihood of developing side effects because of drug interactions will increase, thereby affecting compliance and therapeutic adherence. Patients and their families may also use food supplements and buy off-the-shelf products from health food shops; these may also interact with prescribed medication, thus causing problems with increased likelihood of side effects.

Many cultural groups use pluralistic approaches and, unless explicitly asked, may choose not to reveal such information with the allopathic physician, thus compounding difficulties in therapeutic engagement. Patients and their families may feel that, if they admit to using traditional medicines, they could be seen as backward or stigmatized. Clinicians must explore such usage very carefully and sensitively try to gather as much information as possible on active components, interactions, and side effects from as many sources as possible.

Clinicians need to avoid stereotypes while prescribing medication. For example, not all south Asians will hand over the responsibility to physicians and may wish to be part of the joint decision-making process. It is worth bearing in mind that not all members from the same culture behave in exactly the same way. Thus a clear understanding of the individual's explanatory models and expectations in therapeutic engagement is increasingly important.

Pharmacodynamics

Pharmacodynamics is the study of the effects that a drug has in an organism. This phenomenon refers to the neurotransmitters, the neurophysiological, behavioural, psychological, and social effects of drugs, and their mechanisms of action. Individuals from different cultures show different enzyme changes leading to variable therapeutic responses. Enzymatic differences, variable neurotransmitter systems, and social and psychological differences across cultures all play a role in influencing the pharmacodynamics of a medication, whether it is prescribed or not. Social and healthcare system variations, such as access to drug level assessments, will help to identify potential problems. Individuals who are diagnosed as rapid metabolizers may require higher than recommended doses of medication, whereas those who are slow metabolizers may need lower than recommended doses.

Pharmacokinetics

Pharmacokinetics is the study of how a biological organism affects the fate and the distribution of a drug. This process is affected by absorption of the drug, distribution of the drug, its metabolism, and its excretion. The process of metabolism also reflects cross-cultural and cross-ethnic differences. Body mass index (BMI), body fat, gastric acidity, and other factors, including smoking, will play a role in influencing pharmacokinetics of drugs.

Enzymes

The four enzymes related to CYP450 are found in large numbers in the liver and the gut as well as in the brain, and their polymorphic expression is shown to be associated with personality traits and leading to side effects such as parkinsonism and tardive dyskinesia. These enzymes have also been implicated in an increased risk for various malignancies and autoimmune conditions (Henderson and Vincenzi, 2015). Genetic polymorphisms within genes encoding proteins/enzymes involved in neurotransmitter synthesis, reception, transport, and degradation have been associated with variations in psychotropic drug response (Ng and Bousman, 2018). It is entirely possible that an excess of polymorphism and its impact on enzymes will also influence how fast or slow is the metabolism of a drug. Therefore doses of medication will need to be moderated carefully.

Figure 6.1 illustrates the links between culture and response to drugs.

Table 6.1 illustrates some of the characteristics of the four (of seven) CYP450 enzymes that are important in psychiatry.

CYP2D6 is one of the most important CYP450 enzymes in psychiatry because it is the major metabolic pathway for many psychotropic drugs and is responsible for drug–drug interaction. It also happens to be polymorphic with over 30 mutations (Pollock et al., 1991). Thus, depending upon the population, individuals can be poor metabolizers, immediate metabolizers, extensive, and ultra-rapid metabolizers. Many of the mutations are ethnic-specific (see Henderson and Vincenzi, 2015, for detailed discussion). These metabolic types affect metabolic rates that in turn influence plasma levels and consequently cause side effects and drug interactions. The number of ultra-rapid metabolizers with duplicated genes is low among Swedes,

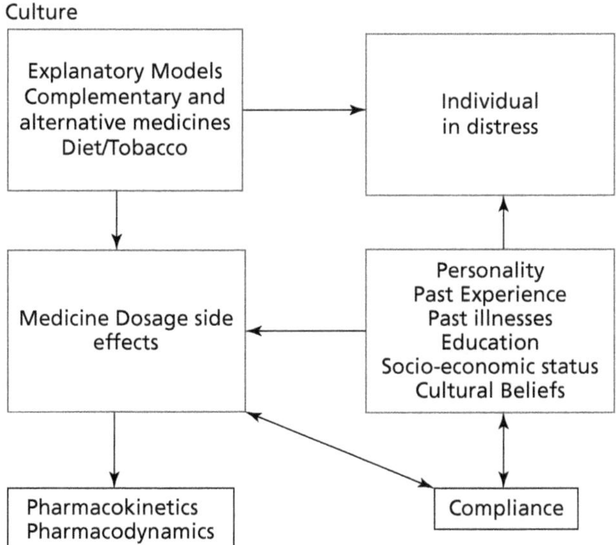

Figure 6.1 Interaction between individual and cultural factors.

Table 6.1 Enzyme substrates and medications affected

Enzyme	Antidepressants affected	Antipsychotics affected	Others
CYP2D6	Tricyclic antidepressants	First-generation neuroleptics	Codeine
	Mirtazapine	Risperidone	Propranolol
	Venlafaxine	Clozapine	
		Olanzapine	
CYP3A4	Selective serotonin reuptake inhibitors	Both second- and first-generation	Mood stabilizers
			Antibiotics
			Antifungals
			Alprazolam
CYP1A2	Tricyclic antidepressants	Second-generation	Caffeine
	Selective serotonin reuptake inhibitors	Clozapine	Propranolol
CYP2C19	Tricyclic antidepressants	Clozapine	Benzodiazepines

American Whites, and Spaniards (Agundez et al., 1995) but high in Arabs (McLellan et al., 1997) and in Ethiopians (Akillu et al., 1996). Thus, those with high ultra-rapid metabolism respond poorly and may be thought of as non-compliant. CYP3A4 enzyme is most abundant in liver and is responsible for biotransformation of a large number of psychotropic medications as well as many other drugs. Some diet and herbal interactions, such as grapefruit and St John's Wort, can cause induction of substrates. Many ethnic groups show low levels.

CYP1A2 is responsible for metabolizing many drugs, including fluvoxamine, haloperidol, olanzapine, etc. Cruciferous vegetables such as broccoli, cabbage, Brussels sprouts, tobacco, and a diet high in protein can induce it (Ionnides, 1999) and, again, ethnic variations have been reported. Smoking can reduce the effectiveness of medications such as clozapine, haloperidol, and olanzapine, and any abrupt changes may produce increased side effects.

CYP2C19 significantly influences the biological transformations of some of the commonly used medications, especially benzodiazepines and some of the selective serotonin reuptake inhibitor antidepressants. East Asians are poor metabolizers compared with whites.

It is apparent that there are clear variations in metabolizing enzymes and their distributions among various ethnic and cultural groups. When clinicians have access to facilities they should have the metabolism of their patients ascertained so that dosages of medications can be titrated. This is especially important in individuals who may be developing side effects and/ or not responding.

Several environmental factors are involved in mediation of CYP450 environmental interactions. Apart from smoking and diet, substances such as tortilla and corn can also cause changes in metabolism. Associated substance abuse can also contribute to changes in metabolism, leading to higher levels of side effects in some individuals. It is possible to obtain a profile of CYP450, although laboratory availability is patchy and not uniform. When this is available, it may be too expensive. High-carbohydrate and high-protein diets can also cause inhibition of some enzymes, thereby leading to problems. Clinicians should routinely enquire about dietary patterns, including dietary supplements, as well as the use of alternative and complementary medicines.

In addition to dietary patterns, dietary supplements, etc., it is also essential that clinicians explore smoking and drinking habits as well as religious and dietary taboos. The use of cola drinks, tea and coffee, and resulting caffeine intake, may also interfere with actions of drugs. Low levels of smoking in some ethnic groups may produce higher levels of plasma levels of medication, especially if individuals also happen to be slow metabolizers. For example, two key interethnic metabolic differences in response to caffeine are genetic acetylator status, which influences levels of paraxanthine (the main metabolite of caffeine) and the urinary metabolism of paraxanthine (Kalow, 1986a, b); there are diverse abilities for recognizing the taste of phenylthiocarbamide across ethnic groups. Tasting ability has also been associated with development of thyroid disease. In addition, levels of drug binding and their transport across the blood–brain barrier also need to be remembered, as these too vary across different ethnic groups. Box 6.2 suggests how pharmacotherapy should be planned.

Medication remains an important part of the therapeutic armamentarium, and the clinician must prepare the patient and their carers and families with the right information and ensure that they understand the meaning of the medication and its purpose and side effects. Cultural variations in explanatory models and the perceived role of the medicine and ethnic variations have to be seen as an essential part of the development of therapeutic intervention. Culturally based health beliefs and treatment options can have a

Box 6.2 Planning pharmacotherapy

Prior to prescribing:

- Check weight/height/body mass index
- Check diet and dietary taboos
- Check religious taboos
- Check complementary/alternative and over-the-counter medications
- Check alcohol, caffeine, nicotine use, and intake
- Check metabolizer intake status if possible

While prescribing:

- Start at lowest possible dose
- Low threshold for identifying side effects
- Adjust dosage slowly
- Provide as much information as possible, including written information to patient and family

After prescribing:

- Monitor side effects regularly
- Train staff, carers, and patient to identify side effects
- Check compliance using serum levels if possible
- Check changes in diet/meds./alcohol/caffeine, etc.

major impact on therapeutic adherence and alliance (Lin and Smith, 2000). Additional factors that must be remembered include subjective experiences of medication rather than direct pharmacological effects, and these are significant in engaging patients (Ng and Bousman, 2018). Negative experiences, not surprisingly, will lead to poor compliance (Awad et al., 1995; Ng and Klimidis, 2008). The impact of culturally influenced attitudes deserves detailed attention in future pharmacological research.

Prescribing factors

Depending upon the type of healthcare system, patients and their families may carry different expectations. For example, in private healthcare systems anecdotal evidence suggests that patients expect quicker recovery and may shop around for doctors who in turn may use polypharmacy to get quicker results. Prescribing habits may well be more important than actual differences in response (Frackiewicz et al., 1997). More qualitative work is required to understand these differences.

Dosages of antipsychotics

The recommended mean daily doses of antipsychotics are lower for Chinese American patients compared with white Caucasian American patients (even after differences in body weight have been taken into account) (Chiu et al., 1992). After matching Asian American and Caucasian American patients on a number of parameters (such as duration of illness, age, and past antipsychotic exposure), Lin et al. (1995) demonstrated that Asian American patients needed lower dosages of antipsychotic medication to control symptoms. One of the major side effects of antipsychotic drugs is tardive dyskinesia, which can be notoriously difficult to treat. Thus, preventing the condition is the most sensible therapeutic strategy. It has been demonstrated that rates of tardive dyskinesia were lower in China in comparison with those in Japan (Pi et al., 1993), thus indicating that there may be multiple factors responsible for variation of rates. In many countries, such as Japan, smaller starting doses of antipsychotics are recommended.

For haloperidol, it is recommended that Asian patients be started on low doses. It has also been shown that Hispanic Americans need lower doses of clozapine and risperidone, whereas for chlorpromazine similar levels (to that of Caucasian Americans) are used. African Americans require lower doses of fluphenazine but higher doses of trifluoperazine in comparison to Caucasian Americans (Gaw, 2001).

As there are ethnic and racial variations in metabolism, different doses are needed for different populations and cultural groups, especially if side effects are to be avoided and optimal responses obtained. However, many drug trials continue to exclude ethnic groups other than white Caucasian groups, thereby making generalizability of findings much more problematic. As a result, similar doses are recommended, leading to higher than expected levels of side effects. Therefore, it is important that clinicians look at individual cultural groups and ethnic differences when deciding what medication to give and what the ideal doses should be, bearing in mind that lower than recommended doses may be required.

Dosages of antidepressants

Owing to variations in pharmacodynamics, pharmacokinetics, and pharmacogenomics, responses to antidepressants also vary across different ethnic groups. As noted earlier, enzyme differences in ethnic groups can cause rapid or poor metabolism of antidepressants. Asians have been shown to metabolize tricyclic antidepressants more slowly and therefore develop more side effects on similar dosages. Caucasian Americans, on the other hand, show rapid metabolization and attain peak plasma levels later in comparison to Asians. The existing data on newer antidepressants and ethnic variations are scanty, although similar variations are entirely possible. Thus, clinicians are advised to start with the lowest dose, monitor side effects very carefully and closely, and increase doses gradually.

In many cultures, polypharmacy is practised as a matter of routine. However, it is important that addition of other medications or compounds may need to be thought through very carefully because of potential drug interactions and the increased likelihood of side effects. A close consideration of pharmacogenetic, pharmacodynamic, and pharmacokinetic factors will enable the clinician to optimize dosage, reduce the likelihood of side effects, and potentially gain better therapeutic engagement.

Benzodiazepines

As noted in Table 6.1, ethnic variations because of enzyme changes and differences in response to benzodiazepines have been observed. The rates of metabolism of drugs like alprazolam and diazepam are said to be slower among Asians, and genetic factors may be more important in explaining these variations (Lin et al., 1995). Similarly, African Americans may also have an increased clearance of other benzodiazepines.

Lithium and mood stabilizers

Racial and ethnic variations in red blood cell sodium and lithium levels were noted over 30 years ago (Westermeyer, 1989) and yet often the same doses are recommended and used in clinical settings. Among Japanese patients, lithium has been shown to be effective at lower dosages; among Taiwanese patients higher dosages have been required, yet they need lower dosages in comparison with American patients (Chang et al., 1984, 1985). In spite of no pharmacokinetic differences, Taiwanese patients require serum lithium levels of 0.5–0.7 mEq/L whereas Japanese and Chinese patients require higher serum lithium levels. Hot weather, dehydration, and religious fasting may all contribute to higher serum levels of lithium. Climate can play a major role, so advice to patients and their carers and families about hydration becomes very significant. Similarly, care must be taken when commencing individuals on other mood stabilizers (such as carbamazepine, sodium valproate, and others) as ethnic variations in metabolism and excretion are likely to influence levels of side effects (also see Ng et al., 2008; Ng and Bousman, 2018).

Non-compliance

Compliance with medication depends upon a number of other social and cultural factors. The most useful of these is the role that medication is seen to play or expected to play in getting the patient better. These expectations allow a better alliance and engagement with medication, particularly if doctors' expectations match those of the patient. Many psychiatric conditions are chronic and may require long-term medication. In some healthcare systems, the availability of medication may be limited due to cost. The actual cost of drugs, along with their expected, perceived, or real efficacy will play a role in compliance. Anecdotally, it has been observed that in some countries patients can only afford medication one day at a time. Thus, regular taking of medication may itself prove difficult. Although information about the medication is given in various forms to the individual, the stress of the clinic itself may not allow thorough understanding of issues. Furthermore, patients and their family members may forget the information, so supplementary written information in simple language should be provided and made easily available. Sometimes going through a long list of side effects may put patients and their carers off the idea of the medication. Increasingly, in many settings patients will bring with them information that they may have gathered from the internet so a clear dialogue is necessary. Clinical judgement is essential to explain the risk/benefits of the medication. Supportive or motivational psychotherapy may enable clinicians to convince the patient of the usefulness and need of the medication. It is important, therefore, to understand the explanatory models held by the patients and their carers. Involving suitable family members in engaging with working with the patient and their education about their illness and role of medication may pay dividends in the end.

Non-biological factors

Several non-biological factors play a major role in influencing drug interactions as well as metabolism of medication. For example, a specific effect of certain food additives or spices must be taken into account. These include substances such as black pepper, garlic, green tea, kava, mace, nutmeg, cinnamon, sage, turmeric, and white pepper, which have been shown to

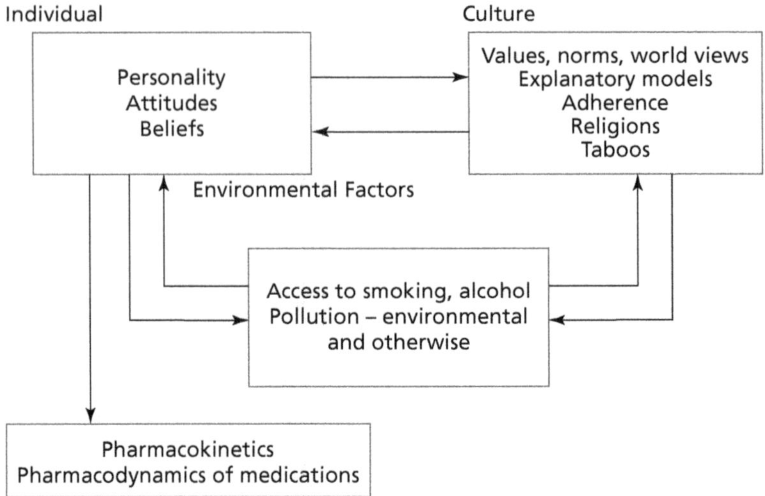

Figure 6.2 Interrelating factors.

cause inhibition of various enzymes, thereby affecting their metabolism and increasing side effects (Henderson and Vincenzi, 2015). Therefore, it is critical that clinicians are aware of dietary habits and advise patients and their carers and families accordingly.

Individual, cultural, and environmental factors affect pharmacodynamics and pharmacokinetics of drugs. Cultures allow or prohibit their members to express their distress or veer too far away from the cultural norms. How individuals see their illness and consequently who they seek help from is strongly culturally influenced. Geographical and financial access to therapists and clinicians will play a major role in who is approached first. This initial clinical contact and subsequent experience and satisfaction with the contact will affect their help-seeking, their models, their therapeutic adherence, and therapeutic alliance. Previous experiences with medication or clinicians and the health services will influence therapeutic engagement.

The interaction of the individual, cultural, and other environmental factors are illustrated in Figure 6.2. These interactions can be very complex in causing changes in therapeutic engagement.

Implementing the treatment plan

Having collected thorough information and mental state assessment with physical investigations as needed, the clinician may reach a clinical diagnosis. The first step is to convey this diagnosis or the differential diagnosis to patients and their carers. The implementation and elements of a pharmacological treatment plan are shown in Box 6.1 and Box 6.2. It is important that patients and their carers are aware of the diagnosis (bearing in mind the issues of confidentiality), the need for treatment, type of treatment needed, potential outcomes, their expectations, and the realities of the intervention. Written information about the illness and therapeutic interventions should be provided in as simple a language as possible. Clinicians should make ample time available to allow patients and their families to ask questions and have their concerns met. If the clinician is not able to do this, every effort must be made to get staff members or others (who are trained to share this information, e.g. the pharmacist) to do so with the family. Sometimes patients or families may present with information downloaded from the internet and, on occasion, this information may be incomplete or incorrect, so clinicians need to be sensitive and aware and avoid patronizing patients and their families.

Conclusions

The clinician must work with patients and their carers as well as families to ensure that patients are taking their medication as prescribed, in the recommended dosages, and correctly. Regular follow-up, monitoring, and available and ongoing discussions about the need for treatment or when and how treatment should be stopped are important steps. The impact of lifestyle, dietary factors, and other biological and non-biological factors must be ascertained clearly and form part of the initial and ongoing assessment. Clinicians must be flexible in tailoring medication according to individual factors within the cultural context. Evidence-based prescription of the right medication in the right dose is important in improving patient outcomes.

References

Agundez J, Ledesma MC, Ladero J, et al. (1995). Prevalence of CYP2D6 gene duplication and its repercussions in the oxidative phenotype in a white population. *Clin Pharmacol Ther*, **57**, 265–269.

Akillu E, Persson I, Bertilsson, et al. (1996). Frequent distribution of ultra rapid metabolisers of debrisoquine in an Ethopian population carrying duplicated and multi-duplicated functional CYP2D6 alleles. *J Pharmac Exp Ther*, **278**, 441–446.

Awad AG, Hogan TP, Vorugunti LNP, Heslegrave RJ (1995). Patients' subjective experiences on antipsychotic medication: implications for outcome and quality of life. *Int Clin Psychopharmacol*, **10** (Suppl. 3), 123–132.

Bhugra D, Ventriglio A (2015). Do cultures influence placebo response? *Acta Psych Scand*, **132**(4), 227–230.

Buckalew LW, Coffield K (1982). Drug expectations associated with perceptual characteristics: ethnic factors. *Percept Mot Skills*, **55**, 915–918.

Chang SS, Pandey GN, Zhang MY, Ku NF, Davis JM (1984, May). *Racial Differences in Plasma and RBC Lithium Levels*. Continuing Medical Education Syllabus and Scientific Proceedings (pp. 239–240). 137th Annual Meeting of the American Psychiatric Association. San Francisco: American Psychiatric Association.

Chang SS, Pandey GN, Yang YY, Yeh EK, Davis JM (1985, May). *Lithium Pharmacokinetics: Inter-Racial Comparison*. Paper presented at the 138th Annual Meeting of the American Psychiatric Association. Dallas: American Psychiatric Association.

Chiu H, Sham P, Lau J, et al. (1992). Prevalence of tardive dyskinesia, tardive dystonia and respiratory dyskinesia in Chinese psychiatric patients in Hong Kong. *Am J Psych*, **149**, 1081–1085.

Frackiewicz E, Stanmed J, Herrara J, et al. (1997). Ethnicity and antipsychotic response. *Ann Psychopharmac*, **31**, 1360–1369.

Gaw AC (2001). *Cross-Cultural Psychiatry*. Washington, DC: APP.

Henderson D, Vincenzi B (2015). Ethnopsychopharmacology. In: RF Lim (ed.). *Clinical Manual of Cultural Psychiatry*. Washington, DC: APA Press, pp. 435–467.

Ionnides C (1999). Effect of diet and nutrition on the expression of cytochrome P450. *Xenobiotica*, **29**, 109–154.

Kalow W (1986a). Caffeine and other drugs. In: W Kalow, H Goedde, D Agarwal (eds). *Progress in Clinical and Biological Research*. New York: Alan Liss, pp. 331–341.

Kalow W (1986b). Outlook of a pharmacologist. In: W Kalow, H Goedde, D Agarwal (eds). *Progress in Clinical and Biological Research*. New York: Alan Liss, pp. 3–7.

Lin K-M (1996). Psychopharmacology in cross-cultural psychiatry. *Mt Sinai J Med*, **63**, 283–284.

Lin K-M, Poland R, Anderson D (1995). Psychopharmacology, ethnicity and culture. *Transcult Psych Res Rev*, **32**, 3–40.

Lin K-M, Smith MW (2000). Psychopharmacotherapy in the context of culture and ethnicity. In: P Ruiz (ed). *Ethnicity and Psychopharmacology*. Washington, DC: APA, pp. 1–36.

McLellan RA, Oscarson M, Seidegard J, et al. (1997). Frequent occurrence of CYP2D6 gene duplication in Saudi Arabians. *Pharmacogenetics*, **7**, 187–191.

Ng CH, Bousman C (2018). Cross-cultural psychopharmacotherapy. In: D Bhugra and K Bhui (eds). *Textbook of Cultural Psychiatry*, 2nd edn. Cambridge: Cambridge University Press, pp. 432–441.

Ng C, **Klimidis** S (2008). Cultural factors and the use of psychotropic medication. In: CH Ng, KM Lin, B Singh, E Chiu (eds). *Ethno-Psychopharmacology: Advances in Current Practice*. New York: Cambridge University Press, pp. 123–134.

Ng C, **Scweitzer** I, **Norman** T, **Easteal** S (2004). The emerging role of pharmacogenetics: implications for clinical psychiatry. *Aus New Zeal J Psych*, **38**, 483–489.

Ng CH, **Lin** KM, **Singh** B, **Chiu** E (2008). *Ethno-Psychopharmacology*. New York: Cambridge University Press.

Pi EH, **Guttirez** M, **Gray** G (1993). Tardive dyskinesia: cross-cultural perspectives. In: K-M Lin, R Poland, G Nakasaki (eds). *Psychopharmacology and Psychobiology of Ethnicity*. Washington, DC: APA Press, pp. 153–168.

Pollock BG, **Perel** J, **Kirshner** M, et al. (1991). 5-mephenytoin 4-hydroxylation in older Americans. *Eur J Clin Pharmac*, **70**, 609–611.

Smith M, **Lin** K-M, **Mendoza** R (1993). 'Non-biological' issues affecting psychopharmacotherapy: cultural considerations. In: K-M Lin, R Poland, G Nakasaki (eds). *Psychopharmacology and Psychobiology of Ethnicity*. Washington, DC: APA Press, pp. 37–58.

Westermeyer J (1989). *Psychiatric Care of Migrants: A Clinical Guide*. Washington DC: APA Press.

Chapter 7

Psychotherapy: General principles

Introduction

Psychotherapy is defined as a process of treatment based on principles of one or more therapeutic schools; the underlying principles are of bringing about sustained individual change using human relationships. Such a change in behaviour or attitudes or the world view starts in therapy sessions and continues even after therapy has been completed. These changes may start in the first therapy session but the work continues outside the therapy sessions, when the patient may start to make connections and sense of what they are experiencing and what they may be going through. Psychotherapy carries different meanings in different cultures, and for some is an alien or unfamiliar experience or cultural practice. Even in high-income countries, people living in deprived inner city areas or those who lack educational opportunities may find a talking therapy difficult and unhelpful. In settings where the specialist is seen as someone wise, the role of therapy may well be very different. The expectations of therapy will also vary. In some cultures, modifying therapy through the use of religious, spiritual, or cultural symbols and aspirations may well be seen as worthwhile.

The role of the therapist

A major responsibility for the therapist is to understand and explore the issues and work with the patient to decide what is needed and how this will be taken forward using the most suitable therapy. A therapeutic alliance is associated with the best outcomes, and this relies on agreeing the common goals, assignment of tasks, and the development of bonds (Bordin, 1979). At an early stage, a clear purpose of the therapy should be explained. Both parties need to understand and agree with this. Mutually agreed goals should be set and clearly stated within the context of cultural expectations as well as the perceived expectations of the family and of society at large.

The proposed goals are those to which both sides commit themselves and may be related to dysfunction focused on one or more individuals. Tantam (2018) suggests that focusing on therapeutic ruptures may be important. Congruence of values between the patient and the therapist, needless to say, will determine therapeutic alliance. Individual and cultural values will both provide a roadmap for the therapist and the patient to work together. Ethnic matching between the patient and the therapist can certainly improve initial engagement, but may not provide better outcomes in the long run. Karlsson (2005) found that there was little evidence that ethnic matching led to better outcomes or greater satisfaction with psychotherapy. Tantam (2018) proposes that this may well be because of the nature of therapy, where patients adjust in response to the therapist, but the question of initial engagement remains.

Types of psychotherapy

Tantam and Sayar (2018) observe that Western psychotherapists and psychotherapy typically draw on two cultural traditions, intertwined within what is called Western European thought, which are to do with explanation and meaning. These authors highlight that the narrative approach to psychotherapy and positivist approaches exist. The religious healing and understanding and what Tantam and Sayar (2018) call unglueing the past are important aspects of psychotherapy.

Wolberg (1967) divides types of psychotherapy into three types: supportive, re-educative, and reconstructive.

1. *Supportive:* in psychiatric care virtually every patient will receive some form of supportive therapy as well as some information and education about the illness, treatment, and outcomes. Supportive therapy provides support during periods of acute stress or in chronic illness when a basic change may not be a realistic goal.

2. *Re-education*: these types of psychotherapy are aimed at remodelling the patient's world view and thinking, with resulting change in behaviour through a focus on promotion and development of new behaviours and causation. Cognitive behaviour therapy and behavioural therapy are re-educative types.

3. *Constructive* therapy aims to change irrational impulses and bring them under control while enabling the individual to develop better coping strategies; these include psychoanalytic and interpretive psychotherapies. Reparative therapy is another form where attempts are made to repair childhood trauma.

There may be some differences between psychotherapy and psychological treatments. Psychological treatments may be behaviour treatments for specific phobias, whereas psychotherapies may be more general. Psychological treatments may be short, focused, and limited in duration, whereas some forms of psychotherapy may take years.

Across cultures, a potential major problem with psychological treatments in general and psychotherapies in particular is that these are based on Western ego-based models, which may not always be easily accepted in other cultures. These approaches may be seen as inappropriate, even threatening, and intrusive to the individual and their families, and unacceptable in their cultural context. In cultures that are sociocentric in which the individual self is embedded in the family or kinship, then egocentric therapies may not be accepted easily. If individuals do not understand or agree with the rationale of psychotherapy, their motivation may become poor and they may find such therapies and interventions unacceptable. Furthermore, if not embedded in the cultural values of the individual, the quality of therapy (no matter how good it is) may not be easily acceptable and therefore it may not lead to therapeutic engagement and consequently may not make any difference whatsoever. In addition, if therapists insist on finding commonality between themselves and patients where none may exist, there will be further tensions in the therapeutic relationship. Psychology too has to be aware of cultural relativism.

Psychotherapy versus shamanist therapies

Shamanist or folk healing practices use cognitive restructuring of meaning in the mind of the patient to control emotional distress and alleviate symptoms (Castillo, 2001). The perceived effectiveness of the healer's methods in the mind of the patient is what Frank (1975) terms the 'expectant faith effect'. Some of this is related to the creation of a charismatic relationship between the healer and the patient. In sociocentric or traditional cultures such expectations of healers—be they traditional, folk, or allopathic healers—may be high. Faith-based healing is often seen as having a number of advantages. These include a commonality of explanatory models but also ease of access compared with professional sectors. Furthermore, there is also a reputational matter here that will attract individuals and their families. A recent study from Western India has demonstrated that it is possible for the professional sector to work with faith healers to improve engagement and outcomes (Shields et al., 2016).

The expectant faith effect has been defined as symbolic healing, which refers to the use of healing symbols (treatments, ritual objects, and placebos) in the healing practice (Dow, 1986). The folk healer may use patients' cultural schema, which are relevant to the illness, and interpret the problem accordingly. These symbols can be both instrumental (with direct physical effect) and purely symbolic (psychological). Religious healing, using religious texts or rituals as well as basic principles derived from other traditions such as Buddhism, can play a major role in moving people to where they need to be. What people read or follow and what they accept are strongly subjected to cultural shifts (Tantam and Sayar, 2018). The therapist must explore the role of religion and spirituality with patients, i.e. whether this is important to them, how it fits in with their explanatory models, and whether these require further exploration or discussion. Cook and Sims (2018) recommend that clinicians must take into account patients' spiritual needs in the same way that religious leaders should take on psychiatric factors.

In many cultures, specific presentations (be they spirit possession, performance or sexual anxiety, or other symptoms, such as spirit loss) may be treated using shamanist approaches. Clinicians therefore need to be aware of the personal and the 'allocated' (by the patient and their carers) significance of the symptoms so that these cannot only be explored but also be utilized in a constructive manner. The therapist must take into account the significance of various symbols, which will improve therapeutic engagement and adherence. Medication itself thus becomes a symbol and in cultures where patients prefer capsules or liquids, tablets may not be seen as suitable.

Tseng and McDermott (1981) have illustrated the universal elements of psychotherapy (Table 7.1). Forms of psychotherapies remain person-specific and the person is both culture-influenced and remains culture-bound, but the therapies and engagement also remain strongly influenced by cultures. The need for conformity will determine what is seen as normal or deviant. The therapist–patient relationship can be both comforting and confronting, and the relevant weight given to either will depend upon the therapist and the type of therapy as well as the patient and their expectations of therapy. Mutual expectations between the therapist and the patient will affect motivation and therapeutic engagement. In many cultures, talking therapies are seen as a waste of time, whereas medication is readily accepted, while in many others it is seen as essential that one has a specialist therapist. These are also likely to be strongly influenced by educational and economic status. Tseng and McDermott (1981) go on to propose that following a thorough assessment, in collaboration with the patient, the clinician identifies the problems and goes on to prescribe appropriate therapeutic intervention. Any prescription for change has to be in the context of

Table 7.1 Steps and components of psychotherapy

Category	Elements
Basic assessment through history	Joint clarification of problems
	Explore cultural factors, explanatory models and expectations
	Agreement on intervention
	Commence therapy with outcomes agreed
Elements of therapy	Cultural transference
	Cultural countertransference
	Unconscious bias
	Racial and ethnic biases
	Comprehensively exploring the problem and agreeing on priorities
	Exploring individual significance
	Type of therapy
Therapeutic outcomes	Social functioning?
	Individual symptom reduction
Termination	Ascertaining needs for termination
Follow-up	Sustainability of changes?
	Recurrence of problems?

the patient's explanatory models and expectations. The therapist needs to understand the causative and perpetuating factors, and work with and encourage the patient to work on these in a culturally appropriate manner. The emotional needs of the patient should be explored and, within the therapeutic parameters, treatment commenced. It is important that both clinician and patient agree on the outcomes and also monitor these throughout the therapeutic process.

A culturally sensitive therapist will not only be aware of cultural differences but also of cultural similarities and the influence of their own culture, and be reflective in their clinical practice. Roles attributed to gender, age, race, culture, and other factors form a part of this attribution and assumptions of therapy. Methods of communication will vary across cultures. For example, issues related to self-disclosure, privacy, and confidentiality will differ, and a good therapist will bear these in mind and take into account all these factors while exploring distress, as well as during treatment planning and therapeutic engagement. The therapist must move away from *a priori* assumptions and utilize cultural knowledge to explore the distress and therapeutic needs of the patient. The power imbalance between the therapist and the patient will vary across cultures, and the clinician needs to take this into account.

Sometimes psychotherapies may need to be modified according to the needs of patients and their cultural models, which may include indigenous therapies that carry specific symbolic meanings. Therapists must therefore be open-minded and reflective in their approaches. The modification may require using multimodal therapies. It is critical that, if using different types of therapies in a modified way, the therapist looks at potential problems before embarking on these.

Language

Both literal and symbolic aspects of language have to be understood and explored in the assessment so that these can be employed successfully in therapy sessions. The use of language, idioms, and expressions is very strongly influenced by culture as well as social and educational factors. It must be recognized that, even when both the therapist and the patient are bicultural and bilingual, the use of language may well vary. Language has to be seen as both a literal expression and as interpretive and nuanced approaches. Furthermore, it is important that the therapist ascertain the preferred language and that it is used correctly. The clinician must also be aware that patients may use language in a defensive or aggressive way. Yamamoto et al. (1993) point out that these switches may reflect a new framework of the meaning (of the word and their experiences). The role of language in psychotherapies is vital and needs better understanding and exploration. The commonality of language is not always feasible, so interpreters may be required to help overcome the barriers of conducting psychotherapy as long as they are not defensive about their cultural norms and values. Interpreters may require a degree of comprehension of psychological concepts, and the interpreter can work as a support worker or cultural broker akin to the surgical nurse supporting the surgeon (Westermeyer, 1989). Linguistic attainment is often one of the first skills to be acquired as part of the acculturative process. Semantic equivalence may occur readily but developing conceptual equivalence may take time. Language can influence non-verbal communication and both need to be ascertained in therapeutic encounters.

Questions about culture

Cultural matters linked with racial and ethnic identity may create a problem. As mentioned earlier, some cultural groups are seen as somatizers (the generation of physical symptoms owing to emotional distress, with an inability to connect the emotional distress to the physical symptoms); they are therefore not seen as responding to psychotherapy so are not offered such treatments.

Occasionally, black and minority ethnic patients or those from minority cultural groups may enter therapy with a pre-existing defence (such as seeing the majority population as the problem), and may thus find it difficult to engage. Ethnic matching of patients and therapists may not always work. Ethnic minority therapists themselves may have experienced a different kind of discrimination, which they may not be willing to share. Also, in spite of their ethnicity there may be a perceived or real power differential between the therapist and the patient. Carter (1995) observes that a person's racial identity may change and, given its close relationship with one's world view and personality, the exact impact of variability of race is not understood. Carter (1995) goes on to raise questions that may need to be explored (Box 7.1). Potential responses to these questions are suggested in Box 7.2.

Racial identity must be explored even when the patient does not see it as an obvious problem. The interaction between the therapist and the patient needs to be ascertained and studied at many levels. As Yakeley et al. (2016) highlight, medical psychotherapy can utilize a mixture of medical and psychological therapies.

Box 7.1 Key questions in psychotherapy

1. Should the question of race be raised and, if so, when?

2. How should the question be framed and raised?

3. What should the therapist do if the meaning and importance of race is denied? Realistic denial?

4. How should poor functioning be differentiated from the impact of race?

5. The ways in which race can affect therapeutic interaction?

Source data from Carter R, *The influence of race and racial identity in psychotherapy: towards a racially inclusive model*, 1995, Wiley.

> ## Box 7.2 Possible answers to key questions in psychotherapy
>
> 1. Race is important and it should be raised as and when necessary.
> 2. The question should be raise in a manner with which the therapist feels comfortable.
> 3. Undue emphasis should not be placed on denial if the patient refuses to explore it in therapy. This may change over time.
> 4. The impact of race should be explored and differentiated from mental state examination.
> 5. Interactional factors must be explored at a number of levels.

Reconstructive therapies

One of the most important reconstructive therapies is psychoanalysis. Psychoanalytic-based psychotherapies have been modified in a number of ways. It is inevitable that, although Freudian principles may be applicable universally, there are huge variations in cultural acceptability as well as acknowledgement of Oedipal complex and child development. The key aim of reconstructive therapies, including psychoanalytic psychotherapy, is to produce long-term change by reducing and controlling impulses and increasing the range and flexibility of psychological defence mechanisms. The basic principle of reparative therapies is the belief that the personality of the individual is dynamic and, through explorations and explanations, these can bring about long-term and sustainable, as well as sustained, changes. The aim is to explore experiences, which may have influenced the individual's childhood and upbringing, and the ways in which these experiences cause problems. Thus, exploration can help to control unhelpful impulses and in learning new coping strategies. The therapist needs special training and personal psychoanalysis and supervision. The phenomena of transference and countertransference emerge from psychoanalysis and are discussed later.

In India, Bose (1949) developed Indian models of psychoanalysis, thus confirming that it is possible to use Freudian principles in other cultures but with suitable caveats. Bose (1949) demonstrated that the Oedipal complex, as seen in the Indian context, varied from the Western context. He observed that the Oedipal complex in India did not work or develop in the same way as it did in Vienna or the West. He argued that the Indian male wanted to castrate his father. The other change was his view about duality, where the conscious and the unconscious were together (Hartnack, 1990).

The three core components of psychoanalysis are free association, interpretation, and transference. The intense nature of the therapeutic relationship creates feelings of transference, exploration of which can lead to an understanding of the reaction that the patient may generate in others as well. In the cultural context, these feelings can be tinged with cultural variations and values, and may lead to further collaboration or rejection of the therapist. Other types of psychoanalysis may thus lead to other specific issues. A challenge for the therapist to work across cultures is to be clear that psychoanalytic psychotherapy focuses by and large on individual functioning and growth, which may be difficult for sociocentric individuals to accept. Furthermore, critique of psychoanalysis from a feminist, sexual orientation, or other perspectives may create specific tensions between the patient and the therapist. Religious or spiritual factors may add another dimension in exploring defence mechanisms. The Oedipal complex and its development in non-nuclear families, along with attachment patterns, must be explored carefully. Sexual thoughts, guilt, and shame across different cultures have varying emphasis and patterns of expression. The phenomena of transference and countertransference will be strongly influenced by a number of factors, and clinicians must be aware of their implications.

Brief dynamic psychotherapy

This is a short, intense, focused treatment dealing with dynamic aspects of pathology and defence mechanisms. The total number of sessions offered typically varies from 10 to 20. The basic aim of such therapy remains building strong therapeutic alliances and helping the patient to work through their specific intrapsychic conflict. Cognitive analytic therapy, for example, is one form of brief psychotherapy that includes dynamic assessment and intervention alongside cognitive and behavioural approaches. The key here is to understand and explore transference and countertransference as well as resistance, along with other defence mechanisms being used by the patient. Underlying levels of motivation can be facilitated to bring about change. These therapies are also influenced by the depth of rapport, the nature of hidden feelings, and the way in which the patient attempts to deal with these. Under certain circumstances such an approach may be better placed in achieving better results with patients from other cultures. Patients from other cultures may not always understand the role of psychodynamic psychotherapy or that of transference, countertransference, or dream analysis. A clear explanation may enable the patient to identify the purpose of such approaches. The expressions of distress and degree of trauma and anxiety experienced may well bring about resistance, which will need to be explored and challenged.

Group therapy

Group therapy brings with it specific challenges, especially in patients from other cultures. Theoretically, it is entirely possible that individuals from sociocentric cultures will be able to work better in groups. Equally plausible is the scenario that they may not wish to share their distress and 'sense of shame' in public. Group therapy can provide insight into social functioning, greater social and self-awareness, and social skills. There is no doubt that the groupwork will be influenced by the theoretical framework practised by the therapist. The number of participants, gender mix, and number of sessions will all be dictated by the purpose of the group. Social skills and social functioning may have different values for different cultural groups. The actual groupwork will be strongly influenced by the purpose perceived by the participants and how motivated they are. Across cultures, psychotherapy may be seen as a Western innovation and groupwork as unhelpful.

Re-educative psychotherapies

Re-educative psychotherapies focus on bringing about relevant changes in behaviour, cognition, or responses to stressors, and the chief aim of such approaches is re-adjustment. Such approaches include behavioural therapies, cognitive behavioural therapies, and humanistic approaches, among others. In certain settings, these may be more appropriate culturally. Thus, individuals may respond more readily as the end results can be seen more clearly and perhaps more readily in fewer sessions. The emphasis in such approaches is to help the individual re-learn habits and attitudes. The focus is not necessarily on regaining insight. Change in behaviour and cognitions may lead individuals to feel that they are gaining self-mastery and an increase in self-esteem.

Behaviour therapy

Cultures will dictate what is abnormal and what is deviant. Therefore, often relatives may determine what they see as abnormal behaviour and whether it is causing distress to the individual or others around them and may require behaviour therapy. In theory, this type of therapy may be more acceptable in some cultures.

Cognitive behavioural therapy

Cognitive behavioural therapy is problem-focused and is thus classified as re-educative. The chief aim of cognitive approaches is to change negative cognitions and develop suitable and appropriate strategies to deal with anxiety, mild depression, and stress, etc. Negative cognitions are caused by the illness and lead to psychiatric symptoms. Cultures affect our cognitions and the way we see the world. Thus in clinical settings, it is important to explore the cognitive schema thoroughly and carefully prior to commencing any therapy. Although it is a Western style therapy, it is possible to modify its approaches to engage patients from other cultures. For example, Beck's cognitive triad includes 'I am a failure', 'the world is a horrible place', and 'my future is bleak'. Thus, the concepts of the self or concept of 'I' will be critical in attempting to change any negative cognitive schema. Similarly, in many cultures, notions of shame will be more prominent than those of guilt in cases of depression. Even within the same culture, notions of guilt or shame will vary. Culture, race, and ethnicity need to be explicitly acknowledged and recognized while planning therapy and its delivery.

Humanistic therapies

These therapies enable patients to develop strategies to achieve self-actualization. The emphasis is on the understanding of what the patient is going through and the process of therapy relies on the therapist's unconditional positive regard, warmth, empathy, and genuineness. These qualities enable the patient to work closely with the therapist. Four key dimensions of transpersonal psychotherapy and approach are critical in engagement: consciousness, conditioning, personality, and identification (Walsh and Vaughan, 1980). Such a model also includes a spiritual dimension, which may be not only useful in many cultures but is also essential so that individuals engage with the therapist.

Supportive therapies

Virtually all patients with physical or psychiatric illness, whether acute or chronic, will need supportive therapy. The psychiatrist does some of the supportive work in regular sessions. For example, while reviewing medication itself the psychiatrist can explore the meanings of medication and side effects as well as point the individual in relevant directions for additional help. Other supportive therapies will include occupational therapy, guidance or milieu therapy, music or art therapies; ventilation, anger management, aids to daily living, etc. The key objective of such therapies is to minimize the impact of a potential threatening event or events. In addition, such approaches can provide support, protection, and relief from responsibility, especially when the patient is going through periods of transition and stress. These approaches can also encourage expressions of feelings and explore theoretical and practical difficulties. These therapies provide an option of supportive work to enable the individual to cope with chronic disabling conditions and can be extremely helpful during times of transition and associated stress. There is every likelihood that such therapies can influence and help individuals to cope better and help them to acquire a level of functioning where more complex and reconstructive therapies can be introduced and long-term changes achieved. The components of supportive psychotherapy include exploration of the problem and the stress; reassurance; explanation; ventilation; guidance suggestion; and support.

Counselling across cultures

In many parts of the world, counselling has become popular and easily accessible, although the quality of counselling is extremely variable. In counselling in general and cross-cultural counselling in particular the key component of the interaction is empathy, and the therapist is both with the client but also separate. Thus, using empathy therapists must accurately reflect feelings and paraphrase or summarize accurately their observations of the behaviour of the individual being counselled. Like all therapies, both verbal and non-verbal communications (which will be very strongly influenced by cultural values and norms) are at the core of the therapeutic interaction.

It is important that patients are aware of the strengths and weaknesses of each therapeutic intervention. It is likely that many individuals will be using indigenous therapies at the same time without informing the therapist, and this may cause problems and give confusing and paradoxical messages to the individuals (Lloyd and Bhugra, 1993; Bhugra and Bhui, 1998).

Conclusions

Interpersonal relationships vary and often result from cultural values and upbringing, and therefore it is critical that these are explored. Both the therapist and the individuals need to be cognisant of verbal nuances as well as non-verbal communication so that there is no room for confusion. The therapist needs not only to explore the underlying dynamics in sessions but to be aware of transference and countertransference, and cultural, racial, or religious elements.

Both parties need to be aware of their own prejudices and conflicts, which must be acknowledged so that they can be confronted and managed. Each type of therapy will have its own issues. For example, group therapy will have different notions and interpretations of various actions in groups depending upon their conscious self and whether it is sociocentric or egocentric and also if the individual feels guilt or public shame and if they are able and willing to acknowledge that in group settings.

If individuals are from a minority culture, as is the therapist, there will be different issues to be negotiated. If there are individuals in the group from varying cultural backgrounds, the dynamics as well as communications will differ. Similarly, couples who hail from different backgrounds may well have difficulties in adjusting with each other but may also have difficulties in communicating with the therapist.

References

Bhugra D, **Bhui** K (1998). Psychotherapy for ethnic minorities: issues, context and practice. *Br J Psychother*, **14**, 310–326.

Bordin E (1979). The generalizability of the psychoanalytic concept of the working alliance. *Psychotherapy: Theory, Research and Practice*, **16**, 252–260.

Bose G (1949). Genesis and adjustment of oedipal wish. *Samiksa*, 3, 237. Reprinted in TG Vaidyanathan, J Kirpal (eds). *Vishnu on Freud's Desk*. New Delhi: Oxford University Press.

Carter R (1995). *The Influence of Race and Racial Identity in Psychotherapy: Towards a Racially Inclusive Model*. New York: Wiley.

Castillo R (2001). Lessons from folk healing practices. In: W-S Tseng, J Streltzer (eds). *Culture and Psychotherapy: A Guide to Clinical Practice*. Washington, DC: APPI, pp. 81–101.

Cook CCH, **Sims** A (2018). Spiritual aspects of management. In: D Bhugra, K Bhui (eds). *Textbook of Cultural Psychiatry*. Cambridge: Cambridge University Press, pp. 472–481.

Dow J (1986). Universal aspects of symbolic healing: a theoretical synthesis. *Am Anthropologist*, **88**, 56–69.

Frank JD (1975). Psychotherapy of bodily disease: an overview. *Psychother Psychosomatics*, **26**, 192–202.

Hartnack C (1990). Vishnu on Freud's desk: psychoanalysis in colonial India. *Social Research*, **57**, 921–947.

Karlsson R (2005). Ethnic matching between therapist and patient in psychotherapy: an overview of findings together with methodological and conceptual issues. *Cultur Divers Ethnic Minor Psychol*, **11**, 113–129.

Lloyd K, **Bhugra** D (1993). Cross cultural aspects of psychotherapy. *Int Rev Psych*, **5**, 291–304.

Shields L, Chauhan A, Bakre R, et al. (2016). How can mental health and faith based practitioners work together? A case study of collaborative mental health in Gujarat, India. *Transcult Psychiatry*, **53**, 368–391.

Tantam D (2018). Therapist–patient relationships and culture. In: D Bhugra, K Bhui (eds). *Textbook of Cultural Psychiatry*. Cambridge: Cambridge University Press, pp. 408–416.

Tantam D, Sayar K (2018). Psychotherapy across cultures. In D Bhugra, K Bhui (eds). *Textbook of Cultural Psychiatry*. Cambridge: Cambridge University Press, pp. 442–457.

Tseng W-S, McDermott J (1981). *Culture, Mind and Therapy: An Introduction to Cultural Psychiatry*. New York: Brunner/Mazel.

Walsh RN, Vaughan EE (1980). *Comparative Models of the Person and Psychotherapy*. Palo Alto, CA: Science and Behaviour Books.

Westermeyer J (1989). *Psychiatric Care of Migrants: A Clinical Guide*. Washington, DC: APA Press.

Wolberg LR (1967). *The Technique of Psychotherapy*. New York: William Heinemann.

Yakeley J, Johnston J, Adshead G, Allison L (2016). *Medical Psychotherapy*. Oxford: Oxford University Press.

Yamamoto J, Silva J, Justice L, Change C, Leong G (1993). Cross-cultural psychotherapy. In: AC Gaw (ed.). *Culture, Ethnicity and Mental Illness*. Washington, DC: APA Press, pp. 101–124.

Chapter 8

Psychotherapy: Specific psychotherapies

Introduction

Cultures carry within them specific languages, and these have specific emphasis on issues related to communicating distress and seeking help, especially if these are seen as talking therapies. The concept of self varies across cultures so any therapy that is trying to re-mould this self must take into account what the type of self within that particular culture is. Additional factors that may play a role in therapeutic engagement in psychotherapy depend upon language, ethnicity, educational, and economic status. That is not to say that poor or uneducated people cannot benefit from psychotherapy—only that different approaches may be needed in exploring cognitions and potential challenges. In many cultures the therapist is seen as sage and wise, like the village elder who can provide wise advice. Expectations are thus influenced by culture. An external locus of control is an important element in explanation in many countries and cultures, and may affect acceptance of therapy as the focus in therapy is on the inner self. The disclosure of emotions to 'strangers' in many cultures can be difficult. Furthermore, disclosure of somatic symptoms to the therapist may cause confusion and problems.

Behaviour therapy

Cultures have a particular impact on psychotherapy, which is especially concerned with meaningful rather than causal connections between events (Tantam and Sayar, 2018).

When a clearly observable behaviour is unacceptable to the individual or to others around them, especially carers and family, then behaviour therapy may be helpful. This therapy may be culturally more acceptable as society and culture determine deviance and behaviours that are deemed to be unacceptable. If such approaches are seen as facilitating and helping individuals to adjust rather than being punitive, they may work better. Older studies showed mixed results with black and minority ethnic populations but, with more experience and better understanding of the culture from which individuals come, therapeutic engagement and outcomes can be improved. Box 8.1 illustrates functional analysis. However, it must also be realized that sometimes this may push psychiatry into being an agent of the state.

In the treatment of phobias, for example, behavioural therapies such as exposure may work better for certain individuals. However, social skills training and assertiveness or anger management training may not be accepted readily in many cultures. In those societies, these may be seen as inappropriate and even unacceptable interventions. Social skills training which prepares an individual to go out on a date may not be acceptable at all in many cultures, especially if they believe in arranged marriage. Thus, there is room for potential misunderstanding and tension between the therapist and family members. Social relationships, social expectations, and environmental norms will depend upon the type of culture from which an individual comes. However, as a result of acculturation these values will change and may even lead to tension between individuals and their carers, especially if their models of explanation vary or if they have different levels of acculturation.

In instituting behaviour therapies, often relaxation techniques are used as the starting point. Again, the method and implications of this will vary across cultures. For example, not all individuals from China will be interested in using tai chi for relaxation and not all Indians will be into meditation or yoga. Thus, an open-minded approach and applying modification to individual understanding will help. Furthermore, as relaxation techniques may be taught as modelling it is important that the patient trusts the therapist. The therapist may need to recruit family members as co-therapists.

Box 8.1 Steps of functional analysis in behaviour therapy

1. Explore and clarify the exact problem
2. Understand individual response and meaning of the problem
3. Assess motivation
4. Analyse steps
5. Social relevance of behaviour
6. Relevant environment in which actions occur

Functional analysis will give a better and clearer picture in setting up behavioural therapy.

Cognitive behavioural therapy

Cognitive behavioural therapy should be seen as problem-focused. The chief aim of cognitive approaches is to change the negative cognitions and develop suitable and appropriate strategies to deal with stress. There is no doubt that an individual's cognitive schema is strongly influenced by their upbringing which in turn is strongly influenced by cultures. In addition, cognitive behaviour therapy should be seen as being strongly culturally influenced, as negative thoughts and concepts of ego may be interpreted in different ways.

In many cultures, going to see a therapist used to be taboo because the therapist was a stranger and discussing personal things with strangers was seen as unacceptable (Oei and Gok, 1998); this has begun to change, and in many countries 'consulting' and counselling have become acceptable and, indeed, fashionable.

The basic components of cognitive therapy are illustrated in Box 8.2. As a re-educative therapy, cognitive work focuses on exploring negative automatic thoughts that individuals may have, and they have to be trained on how to use various techniques to challenge the negative automatic thoughts.

Box 8.2 Steps in cognitive therapy

1. Identify the problems clearly in the context of culture
2. Identify the objective components in a culturally appropriate way
3. Ascertain precipitating and perpetuating factors, including vulnerabilities
4. Explore cognitive schema within the world view
5. Ascertain coping strategies—whether these are culturally appropriate
6. Explore automatic thoughts
7. Set up strategies for challenging negative automatic thoughts; homework based on activity is required
8. Start with what is a manageable and achievable task and build on it
9. Evaluate and modify if needed
10. Teach coping strategies according to cultural values

There is considerable evidence that cognitive behaviour therapy works very well in many conditions, but its success across cultures needs further validation. It is time-limited, focused, and effective. The advantages outweigh the disadvantages. The recent Increasing Access to Psychological Therapies (IAPT, 2012) programme in the UK has relied on training a large number of cognitive behaviour therapists to provide improved and easy access. Homework is important in cognitive behaviour therapy but there may also be problems in application; in some cultures this may be seen as too childish, whereas in other cultures tasks are accepted readily. Cognitive therapies also include behavioural tasks as a key part of the treatment. Thus, individuals have to be both motivated and active participants/partners in therapy.

Supportive therapies

Irrespective of the severity and type of illness, often patients will require some form of emotional support. Depending upon the needs of the individual, specific disciplines may take on the role of providing support, e.g. social worker for social support. In many cultures, bland reassurance from a professional may not be accepted. Social and cultural expectations of the therapy will also play a role. In sociocentric cultures where interdependence is encouraged, the emphasis on independence in this context will not be acceptable. In a similar vein, other therapies (such as music or art therapies) may be seen as superfluous and may not match the expectations of patients as well as those of their carers and families. Equally, they may see occupational therapy as demeaning, beneath their status, and trivial. For example, such approaches in teaching daily living skills may have to be employed carefully. In many cultures in which marriages are arranged, providing social skills when meeting members of the opposite sex may well be seen as pointless. Gender roles and gender role expectations will determine what is seen as acceptable and what is partially acceptable.

Other therapies, such as marital or couple therapy, family therapy, and indigenous therapies, are often needed. It must be remembered that the general principles of psychotherapy across cultures will apply but, for each of these, some additional modifications may be required. Each of these therapies can be reductive, reconstructive, or supportive, or even a mixture of more than one approach (see Yakeley et al., 2016 for details).

Couple and marital therapy

Couple work, whether the couple present with sexual dysfunction or relationship problems or a mixture of both, is strongly influenced by cultural factors. The emergence of such approaches from the systems theory suggests that the relationship in a couple or in the family is likely to be affected by even the most subtle changes in these milieux. The relationship between the couple can be looked at in any number of ways and interventions offered accordingly.

Increasingly, clinicians are likely to come across mixed culture couples and thus need to be aware that some relationship issues will require a better understanding of cultural variations or even culture conflict between the couple but also with the therapist. If the couple come from a different culture from that of the therapist, additional tensions may emerge. Thus the therapist needs to be fully aware of potential problems and pitfalls. The clinician needs to take into account the cultural expectations of the relationship or marriage and must respond accordingly. In some of these settings the therapist may need to take on the mantle of village or family or kinship elder, providing guidance and advice. In sociocentric societies, marriage is often a relationship between two families, with individuals simply representing such connections, as used to be the case in many cultures centuries ago. The style and the contents of therapy will have to reflect such variations, especially if the individuals see sexual activity primarily as for procreative purposes. The couple's world view and their expectations of marriage and therapy must be explored before therapy is commenced. The couple and the therapist must agree on the aims and objectives of therapy before it starts. Thus, the first few sessions should be used to explore needs and develop therapeutic strategies, which will enable the couple to agree to the same goals. Mutual expectations, past experiences, and marital/couple interaction will need careful exploration (Figure 8.1).

Unless the therapist is aware of the cultural biases and nuances, the couple may not engage with therapy. Indeed, it may lead not only to problems in

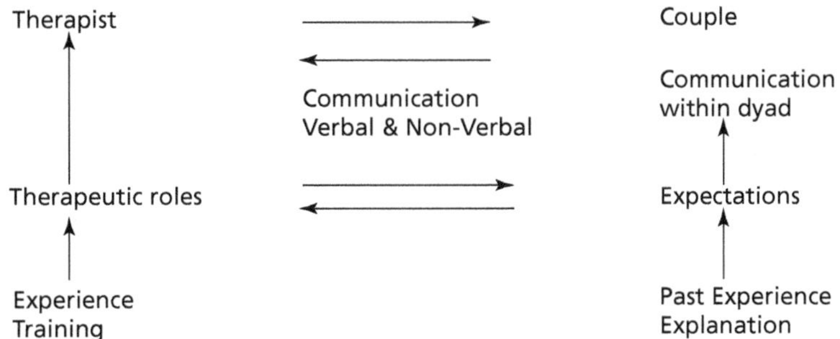

Figure 8.1 The therapeutic relationship in couple therapy.

Box 8.3 Universal elements of therapy

1. Identify and 'name' the problem
2. Explore precipitating causes
3. Explore perpetuating factors
4. Explore explanatory models
5. Explore expectations of therapy
6. Empathy, understanding, and explanation/exploration

---

the therapeutic relationship but may also cause damage to the couple's relationship. Within each mode of psychotherapy being offered it is possible to identify components that may be applicable at a universal level. These are illustrated in Box 8.3. Therapists, if they are not aware (or sufficiently familiar with) of the culture of the couple, may need a longer period of assessment and to create a space to orientate themselves with the cultural mores and values. Exploring and narrowing down the causes of friction and problems through careful dialogue can enable therapists to build strong therapeutic alliances. Some of these factors will apply to the therapeutic interaction even if the couple and the therapist hail from the same culture. Microcultures and microidentities may play an important role in moulding attitudes to sexual activity and relationships, and therefore require clear exploration.

Couples and their therapists

The setting up of therapeutic interaction, assessment, therapy, and agreement on the outcomes will influence the therapeutic alliance and adherence. The couple as a unit may interact with the therapist and create a dyad. The two members of the couple may well have different and varying agendas. Thus, within each therapeutic dyad, the ethnocentrism of the couple and of the therapist, the power imbalance between the couple and the therapist (and within the couple), and alliance with or against the therapist will play a role in therapeutic interaction. This is illustrated in Figure 8.2.

If the therapist and the couple are from different ethnic, racial, or cultural backgrounds, there may be a need to clarify these factors so that any management plans can be made sensitively and sensibly. These interactions are shown in Figure 8.3.

The healing relationship is likely to be influenced by the personality characteristics of the therapist and the couple. Cultural norms and cultural

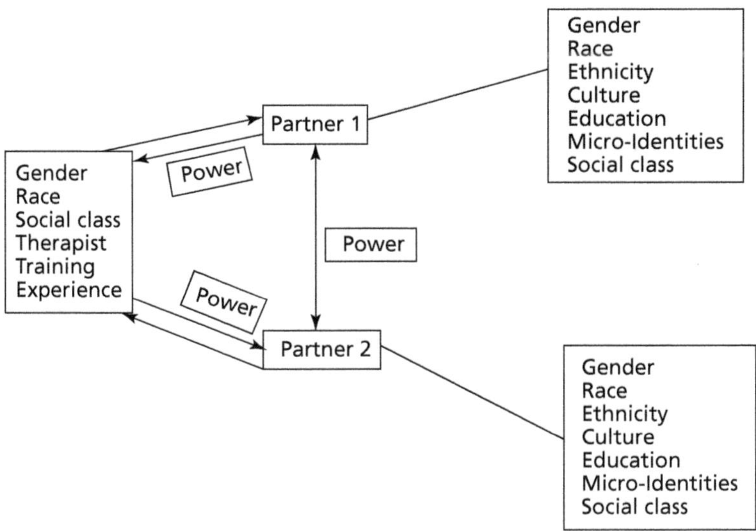

Figure 8.2 The therapeutic relationship and communication.

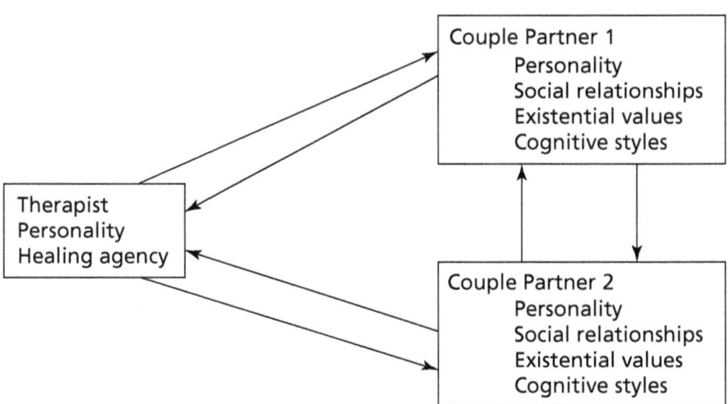

Figure 8.3 Interaction between couple and therapist.

expectations strongly affect the power relationship or the perceived power embedded in the therapist. However, in the case of couple therapy this is further complicated by the expectations of the couple, who may carry varying or competing expectations. Key stages of the couple therapy process are illustrated in Table 8.1.

The power embedded in the therapist is a result of the culture in which they trained and practise, indicating that some couples, or indeed the individuals, may hand over power to the therapist, expecting the therapist to sort out the problems and 'bless' the couple. This perceived power differential may actually place the therapist in a more vulnerable position. It may also 'excuse' the couple, so there must be a clear discussion about the reflections and expectations of the therapy at an early stage.

Concepts of the self will differ depending upon whether both partners in a couple relationship are sociocentric or egocentric. These characteristics of cultures are also likely to affect pathways into care and methods of seeking help. The individual's notions of self and self-image, as well as self-esteem, are important in therapeutic engagement and alliance, and this in itself may create difficulties in couple therapy sessions. Figure 8.4 illustrates the relationship between the therapist and the couple if they hail from different cultures.

In many cultures, couples may live in a joint (extended family all in one house) household with limited privacy and common kitchen and living space. Thus, therapists need to be cognisant of the fact that giving them homework for sexual therapy may not be achievable, and the 'separation' or 'individuation' of the couple may not be entirely possible or indeed even under consideration. The systems approach therefore may offer the most suitable assessment and management strategies. The style and content of

Table 8.1 Stages of couple therapy

Stage	Areas to be tackled
1. Assessment	Problem
	Why here? Why now?
	Cultural norms and expectations
	Verbal/non-verbal communication
2. Engagement	Positive and negative
3. Therapeutic alliance	Transference and countertransference
4. Termination	Outcomes

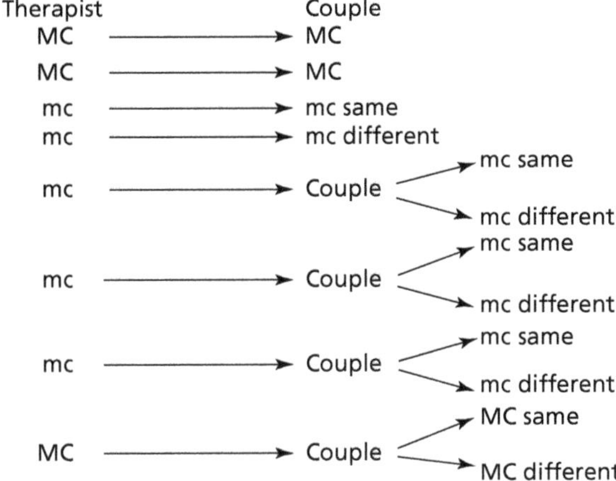

Rarely two therapists may be involved and thus similar dyads will emerge

MC = Majority culture

mc = Minority culture

Figure 8.4 Potential areas of therapeutic interactions.

assessment and management will reflect the relevant cultural values and mores. It is entirely possible in more patriarchal cultures that men may find it difficult to accept that couple therapy is needed, blaming the female partner, and this in itself will affect motivation and help-seeking. Thus, the therapist must be fully aware that in some situations the presenting couple may be reflecting a much larger family issue, whilst not using stereotypes but exploring each couple's unique cultural practices. The therapist must be sensitive to their own weaknesses and strengths as well as to what to expect from the therapeutic encounter. Presenting factors and vulnerability factors are illustrated in Figure 8.5.

The self-awareness of the therapist and key aspects are illustrated in Box 8.4. Assessment of couples in couple therapy is shown in Box 8.5. The cultural norms of each individual within the couple should be explored both separately and together to understand and explore if there are any underlying areas of culture conflict (Box 8.6).

In addition to exploring the why, why now, and why here questions the therapist must strive to explore other factors in assessment at a more focused level. It is important to avoid stereotypes and racial caricatures as a result of underlying prejudice. Cultural norms related to marriage and couple

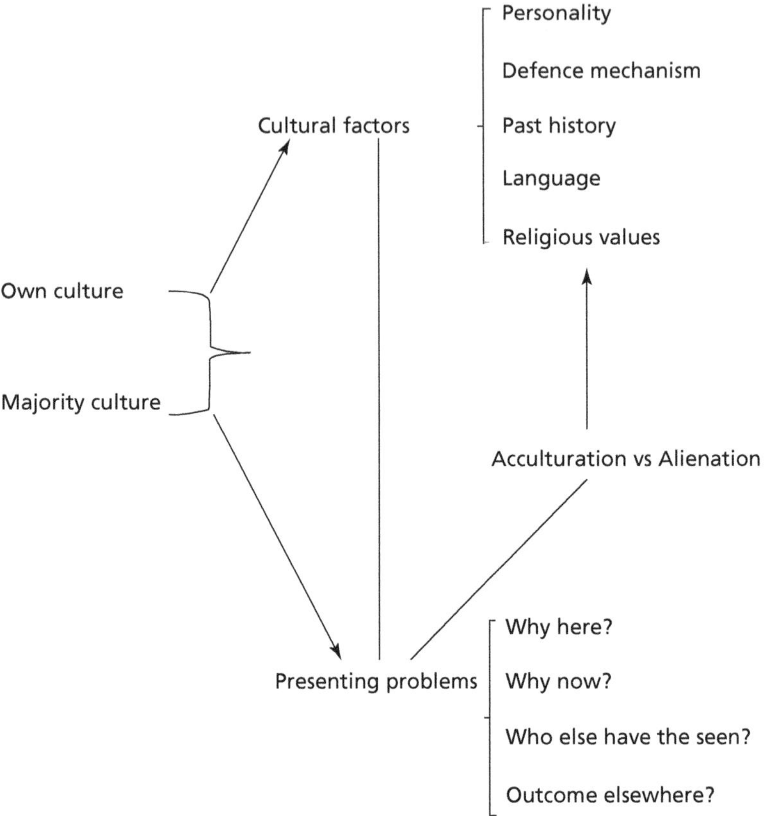

Figure 8.5 Presenting problems and precipitating/vulnerability factors.

Box 8.4 Therapists' strengths and weaknesses

- Be aware of own likes, dislikes, prejudices
- Be aware of self-identity—microidentities and their impact
- Be aware of ethnic and cultural factors affecting own 'world view'
- Be aware of transference and countertransference
- Be sensitive to the possibility of idealizing one or other culture
- Be aware of strengths and weaknesses of own culture as well as of others

Box 8.5 Assessing couples

Assess problem:

- How defined? Who defined it?
- Why here? Why now? Expectations of therapist?
- Cultural emphasis and nuances
- Expectations of each other
- Expectations of therapy

Assess relationship:

- Psychological support
- Financial support
- Children
- Intimacy—emotional and sexual
- Sources of support
- Sources of stress
- Biculturalism
- Issues related to fidelity
- Cultural expectations of the couple

therapy are shown in Box 8.7. These are particularly applicable to individuals whose cultures the therapist may not know.

The assessment must explore the quality of the actual relationship and the personal and social expectations. If the problems are accompanied by sexual dysfunction, for example, then both the dysfunction and the relationship have to be explored at length. The role of sexual activity in the culture must be ascertained—whether the sexual act is seen as a pleasurable (sex-positive) activity or as a purely procreative (sex-negative) act. In addition to exploring the actual quality of the relationship, the therapist must also assess the strengths and weaknesses in the couple relationship. If the couple have cultural differences related to belonging to different ethnicities, these need to be assessed carefully and sensitively. Box 8.8 illustrates potential strengths of interethnic relationships.

In some cases, it is entirely possible that the therapist feels a sense of injustice and may try to jump in with missionary racism. The therapist may, in a paternalistic and patronizing way, decide that they 'know' what is wrong

- Racial issues
- Religion, religious, and spiritual values
- Perceptions of therapy at individual and couple level
- Role and responsibilities within and for family
- Family expectations of the couple
- Language, fluency, and communication
- Ensure that communication is clear and understood
- Discordance, if any, of the self in the couple and expectations of each other
- Ascertain cultural identity
- Cultural, racial, ethnic similarities and differences

- Normative age of marriage in their culture?
- Why that age?
- Role of marriage? Marriages arranged?
- If the couple are not married, what are the cultural expectations of live-in relationships?
- Gender roles in marriage?
- Choice of partner allowed?
- Who takes responsibility for matchmaking?
- Acculturation and continuity of these patterns
- Cultural expectations of mate selection?
- Division of responsibilities?
- Cultural emphasis on reproduction?
- Cultural expectations of reproduction?

Box 8.8 Strengths of interethnic relationships

- More thorough preparation for marriage? Prepared for managing risk
- Degree of commitment? Likely to be greater
- Greater degree of respect, tolerance?
- More accepting of differences?
- More flexibility in relationships?

and that all the problems the couple are facing are related to their race or ethnicity. Thus, the therapist may feel a need to step in to save the couple from themselves. Such feelings of missionary racism are likely to create major issues in both the therapist and in therapy. The therapist may not actually be aware of such interactions and this may contribute to difficulties.

Some of the assumptions that can be potentially problematic are illustrated in Table 8.2. These feelings and responses in relation to therapy may be related to the implicit and explicit power embedded in the therapist. This power, combined with cultural nuances, may well create major problems for both the therapist and the couple (Table 8.3).

Table 8.2 Potentially dangerous assumptions made by the therapist

Type of assumption	Nature of assumption/example
Colour-blind	Assuming that all ethnic minority clients are the same as the majority (ignoring individual experiences)
Colour-conscious	All problems 'blamed' on race
Cultural transference	Patient's feelings are related to the therapist's race
Cultural countertransference	Therapist's feelings toward the patient result from their own race
Cultural identification	Minority therapists overidentify with the patient and see problems as race-based
Identification with oppressor	Minority therapists deny their status by virtue of power

Source data from Ridley CR, *Overcoming Unintentional Racism in Counselling and Therapy*, 1995, SAGE Publications.

Table 8.3 Advantages related to power differentials

Majority culture (MC) and minority culture (mc) participants in therapy	Potential advantages
MC therapist/MC patient	Help reaffirm shared cultural experiences and values
MC therapist/mc patient	Awareness of differences
mc therapist/mc patient	Shared identity and possibly shared experiences
mc therapist/MC patient	Shared learning

MC=Majority client

mc=minority client

Therapeutic interventions

In all cases, there is a need to explore what the couple see as their problems. Occasionally they may feel that they have been misunderstood or they may mistakenly see the problem as abnormal even if it is within the normative range. Such experiences are relatively common when presenting with psychosexual dysfunction. Under these circumstances, education and careful explanation are essential.

The disadvantages of the power differential across the therapist/patient relationship related to ethnic, racial, and cultural differences are illustrated in Table 8.4. Therapists must be aware that they have to both learn and educate their patients and others. Various potential strategies for education are illustrated in Box 8.9.

These advantages and disadvantages may be seen as too generalized, but therapists should be able to understand and respond in a culturally sensitive

Table 8.4 Disadvantages related to power differentials

Majority culture (MC) and minority culture (mc) participants in therapy	Potential disadvantages
MC therapist/MC patient	Potentially lost opportunity to grow
MC therapist/mc patient	Sense of cultural inequality and communication
mc therapist/mc patient	Loss of hope, loss of confidence
mc therapist/MC patient	Poor communication Perceived/real power differential

MC=Majority Client

mc=minority client

> ## Box 8.9 Educational strategies
>
> - Understanding social and cultural differences
> - Clear communication
> - Clear contents—supported by written information
> - Clear language
> - Time for further clarification and discussion

manner. Furthermore, educational strategies must be tailored and not used as a 'one size fits all'.

The educational strategies and psychological nuances will need to be applied very carefully. In some situations, members of minority ethnic groups may be using indigenous therapies at the same time without informing the therapist. Under these circumstances, there is a clear danger that the two types of approaches may give confusing and paradoxical messages to the couple (Lloyd and Bhugra, 1993; Bhugra and Bhui, 1998).

Family therapy

Structures and functions of families will be very strongly influenced by cultures and societies. For many groups, over the generations due to migration and movements from rural to urban areas, the structure of families may change from joint to nuclear. However, in sociocentric cultures, expectations from members of the family may well remain the same and therefore put pressure on individuals. This shift without changes in gender roles or gender role expectations may cause tensions in the couple as well as affect the family functioning.

There is a serious likelihood that the structures that reflect health in Western nuclear families may not accurately represent the differences in joint families. In non-Western traditional cultures enmeshment may be common and seen as non-pathological; however, Western therapists may see this as pathology and be critical, thereby alienating members of the family. It is important that clinicians see these variations and levels of pathology in the context of culture and, if they are not aware of these factors, they must seek advice from community leaders or other sources. It is to be expected that, in sociocentric cultures, especially among sociocentric individuals, family will be the prime source of support as well as tension, and individuals may find it difficult to individuate from the family in the Western sense. In sociocentric or kinship based cultures, mutual dependence, mutual loyalty, and obligations are often seen as the norm, and any attempts to modify these are likely to be met with resistance. When extended families are the norm, these will also represent keen and strong ties of mutual support. It is important not to idealize or pathologize one or another type of family. Key aspects of assessment are illustrated in Box 8.10. In many cultures, especially in response to poverty, illness, or other factors, children may take on roles in which they look after their parents. Family structures and family constellations also change with time and alter the social, familial, and personal obligations and functions.

When faced with unfamiliar structures and constellations, the therapist must clarify from the family as well as other contexts what is pathological or dysfunctional and what is not and should not be taken at face value. Symbolic and real values of individual roles and role expectations in the family context need to be explored and understood clearly, so that the therapist can avoid any confusion.

Culture conflict, especially across generations, may lead to tensions within the family. Younger generation members may identify closely with their majority member peers whereas their parents may stick to older values and traditions. First-generation migrants may make some effort to acculturate and adapt, and second-generation migrants may have a very different world view. The therapist may be seen as belonging to the older generation, and

Box 8.10 Assessing family factors

1. Understand family structure—recent changes, idealized expectations—may need genograms
2. Structures and role when living together
3. What are the normative structures?
4. Clarify gender roles and gender role expectations and responsibilities—expected and real
5. Generational and culture conflict, if any
6. Discrepancies in acculturation among different members—could this be the source of tension and confusion?
7. Identify the conflict between the roles and role expectations of family
8. Linguistic competence and variation
9. World view of members—has it changed due to acculturation?
10. What are their expectations of therapy?

expectations held by the younger generation of the therapeutic encounter should be taken into account while assessing the family for therapy. The feeling of going to a therapist and washing the family dirty linen in public may lead to resistance as well as avoidance. The role of other agencies—perceived or real—may cause further tensions.

Therapeutic interactions between Western schooled therapists and minority families may be stressful. As presentation of the symptoms and the underlying expectations are influenced by cultural factors, any changes in family structures will also affect their expectations of the family authority. Other factors in the majority culture, such as poverty, overcrowding, and racism, will influence attitudes and behaviours. An open and honest acknowledgement of such factors of adversity, even if the therapist is not able to do anything about these, can be a helpful start, giving a clear message to the family that the therapist is aware and sensitive to these factors.

It is important to ascertain the pressures that families from other cultures may feel to conform to the norms of the majority community. Individually fitted psychological roles and expectations can be identified, but such an approach has to look at overall relationships and expectations (perhaps to conform). Apart from the core members, sometimes additional members may be invited to join sessions almost as elder wise people either on an occasional basis, as and when needed, or on a regular basis.

The focus and the goals of therapy should be clear. Identifying, clarifying, and respecting cultural values and norms and the nature of therapy have to be dealt with in a careful manner. Occasionally, and depending upon need, the therapist may need to work with subsystems within the family, respecting boundaries, but it must be made clear to the family that such approaches may be temporary.

A skills-based approach may be used to reduce situational stress and culture conflict. It must be remembered that family members can take on both positive and negative roles in the patient's life. These are illustrated in Box 8.11. These roles are expected to change as the family therapy progresses.

Box 8.11 Role of family members in therapy

- To provide information about the patient and the circumstances
- Work as co-therapists through receiving information and support
- Source of conflict as well as support
- Focus for intervention

Box 8.12 Indications for family therapy

- A problem in the family requiring external input for resolution
- Family's willingness to express their concern and attend
- Family's commitment to therapy
- Problem may be of individuation
- Scapegoating as a result of acculturative processes

Indications for family therapy are illustrated in Box 8.12. The family may present to the therapist for any number of reasons and these are illustrated in Box 8.13. For families with children and adolescents it is inevitable that the focus will be different and, within the family, other family members may require help. Not all members of the family will undergo acculturation at the same rate. Family therapy thus may need to have a varied focus and will require taking different levels of language and acculturation into account.

For ethnic minority families the assessment for family therapy may need additional enquiries and this is illustrated in Box 8.14.

Assessments for family therapy with minority groups are illustrated in Box 8.15. Therapists must make themselves aware of the basics of the culture to which the family belongs. They can collate such information from a number of resources. Acculturation, cultural values, and cultural nuances can be explored during therapy as long as individual members are willing to share their experiences, and often this is the relatively easy part of therapy. Therapists have to be receptive to the idea of expanding their knowledge and willingness to learn.

Box 8.13 Reasons for presenting

- Marital discord reflected by children's dysfunction
- Psychosexual problems
- Help for early intervention
- Understanding childhood disorders
- Understanding individuation, culture conflict, cultural bereavement, and culture shock

> ## Box 8.14 Ethnic minorities' assessments
>
> Check:
>
> - Expectations of their own culture and the majority culture
> - Acculturative processes
> - Effect and impact of racism in different contexts affecting individuals and family
> - Problems in adjustment
> - Culture and external factors, tensions related to sociocentric versus egocentric
> - Culture and internal factors: self-esteem, language, dress, etc.

The family may present the individual as the problem because of culture conflict or varying levels of acculturation, whereas the underlying problems may be more systematic. These goals may also be affected by various other factors, such as socioeconomic status, microidentities of different individuals, and expectations and perceptions of the role of family and the role of marriage. The gender roles within the family system will also be of major importance in therapy. Family expectations of each of the family members and deviation from cultural norms may cause further alienation and difficulties.

When working across cultures, therapists may need to prepare themselves for a number of issues prior to commencing therapy. These are illustrated in Box 8.16. The potential conceptual framework is shown in Box 8.17.

During the therapy itself, there may be specific processes that may prove to be crucial in family engagement and in communicating with the family. Therapists may need to be aware of specific theoretical models and their advantages or disadvantages for specific cultural groups. The extent of acculturation should be ascertained sensitively and carefully without appearing to be patronizing.

Gender roles must be explored along with gender role expectations. These are illustrated as broad guidelines in Box 8.18. In couple therapy as well as in family therapy, the therapist may need to explore the quality of the relationship between not only the principal couple but also other members of the family. Some of these questions are illustrated in Box 8.19. The quality of relationships must be ascertained very sensitively, as in many cultures

Box 8.15 Family therapy: assessment

Preparation:

- Family and cultural values
- Family and kinship structures
- Mate selection
- Child rearing patterns
- Sibling relationships
- Cultural expectations of the family
- Interracial marriages
- Attitudes to divorce
- Impact of migration and acculturation
- Cultural identities—macro and micro

Therapy:

- Communication skills
- Family structure therapy
- Problem-solving phase
- Evaluation of agreed outcomes
- Termination

Some additional factors:

- Time orientation
- Role of extended family
- Preferred mode of action—doing versus becoming

public acknowledgement of difficulties in a relationship is akin to failure and resulting shame. Therapists must be aware of their own 'self' and some of the questions that may help are shown in Box 8.20.

In addition, therapists must also be sensitive to and aware of the impact of racism at an individual as well as at an institutional level on individuals seeking help. Missionary racism is where therapists (in a position of power) may feel that they know what is best for their patients. Such a patronizing position can cause more problems than it solves. Therapists must have a reflexive attitude. They must be able to, as well as willing to, explore therapeutic relationships and learn these interactions and grow.

Box 8.16 Preparing for family therapy

Understand:

- Cultural norms
- Family norms—structure, etc.
- Marriage settings
- Attitudes to marriage as such and to interracial marriages
- Sibling relationship expectations
- Implications if family were to break up
- Cultural identities and levels of acculturation in each individual
- Patterns of distress and help-seeking
- Gender roles and gender role expectations
- Preferred modes of activity: doing versus being

Counselling across cultures

A key aspect of counselling in general and cross-cultural counselling in particular is the role that empathy plays, and the therapist is 'with the client' but also distinct and respectful (Carkhuft, 1969). In the use of empathy, the therapist must take into account an accurate reflection of feeling and paraphrase or summarize accurately the observations. Basic listening skills rely

Box 8.17 Conceptual framework

Check:

- Cultural reality, cultural bereavement, cultural shock, and culture conflict
- Acculturation levels in different members
- Ethnic differences, if any
- Language, self-esteem, attitudes to family, etc.
- Systems in the family
- Reality and expectations of the family members of therapy and of therapist whether they are seen as saviour

Box 8.18 Gender role assessment

- What does being female/male mean to you? To culture?
- How does it affect your role?
- How does it affect others' expectations?
- What does you being female/male mean to your family?
- What do these expectations mean to you and how do they make you feel?
- What will your ideal male/female role be?
- How does your gender affect your relationship and your functioning?
- How do you interpret your family's reactions to you as being due to your gender?

on exploring both verbal and non-verbal communications, which will be very strongly influenced by cultural values and norms.

The first step is establishing rapport and structure for counselling. Then accurate data must be collected to ascertain needs and aims of counselling. An agreed outcome will enable both the therapist and the presenting individual to work together. Alternative solutions and outcomes may have to be explored. Fukuyama (1990) describes a model of transcultural counselling and this is illustrated in Box 8.21.

When working with couples or families using counselling approaches, more than one perspective will have to be explored, understood, and

Box 8.19 Assessment of quality relationship

- Who is your closest confidant? If not, partner/family member—why?
- How open are you about your emotions and feelings with them?
- Are you free to discuss all your problems?
- Are you able to seek and get emotional support? If not, why not?
- What would you like to be different in this relationship?
- Are you able to respond if they seek emotional support?

Box 8.20 Therapists' self-examination

- Are you aware of your cultural values?
- Are you aware of your ethnic heritage?
- Are you aware of your strengths and weaknesses as well as those of your culture?
- Are you monocultural, bicultural, or mixed?
- What message does each culture give you?
- What message from each culture do you give to others?
- How do these messages affect your therapeutic relationships?
- How sensitive are you to discrepancies between your cultural values and those of individuals you are seeing?

employed in treatment. Multilevel or a web of interventions may be needed. The impact of culture cannot be underestimated. Communication within the family will be influenced by cultural values and cultural paradigms. The therapist may need to develop culture-specific and innovative strategies to provide optimal direction.

Box 8.21 Transcultural counselling

- Define culture broadly and microidentities
- Beware of stereotyping
- Understand significance of language and non-verbal communication
- Encourage loyalty and pride to culture
- Ascertain acculturation
- Gender role variations
- Facilitate development of identity
- Strengthen self-esteem
- Explore the world view in the context of culture

Source data from Counselor Education and Supervision, 30, Fukuyama M. Taking a universal approach to multicultural counselling. *Counsellor Education and Supervision*, pp. 6–17, 1990, John Wiley & Sons.

Conclusions

Talking therapies are an integral part of psychiatric practice and it is important that these are culturally appropriate and culturally sensitive. Encouraging both the therapist and the individuals undergoing psychotherapy to explore cultural values will allow both parties to learn about what is helpful and needed and which issues to focus on. Such an approach also avoids overreliance on stereotypes and ensures that person/couple/family subcultures are fully understood before embarking on therapy. Variations in race, culture, language, and ethnicity may well add further complicating factors. Problems in relationships arise from a number of sources, such as incompatibility of personality, mixed motivations, different expectations, and different feelings about relationship and marriage may also be influenced by varying cultural values and cultural world views. Basic universal principles of psychotherapy can be applied as long as the therapist is aware of and sensitive to differences across cultures. It is imperative that clinicians take into account microidentities, which may well be causing tensions and friction not only between individuals but also within the same individual. The key in psychotherapy is learning, and how it is expressed and accepted is critical and is very strongly influenced by culture.

References

Bhugra D, Bhui K (1998). Psychotherapy for ethnic minorities: issues, context and practice. *Br J Psychother*, **14**, 310–326.

Carkhuft R (1969). *Helping and Human Relations*. Vols **1 & 2**. Troy, MO: Holt, Rinehart, and Winston.

Fukuyama M (1990). Taking a universal approach to multicultural counselling. *Counsellor Education and Supervision*, **30**, 6–17.

IAPT (2012). IAPT—three years report: the first million patients. Available online www.iapt.nhs.uk/silo/files/iapt-3-year-report.pdf

Lloyd K, Bhugra D (1993). Cross cultural aspects of psychotherapy. *Int Rev Psych*, **5**, 291–304.

Oei I, Gok Y-W (1998). Issues in the applications of behaviour therapy and constructive behaviour therapy in Asia. In: MTPS Oei (ed.). *Behaviour Therapy and Cognitive Behaviour Therapy in Asia*. Glebe, NSW: Edumedia, pp. 7–14.

Ridley CR (1995). *Overcoming Unintentional Racism in Counselling and Therapy*. Thousand Oaks, CA: Sage.

Tantam D, Sayar K (2018). Psychotherapy across cultures. In: D Bhugra, K Bhui (eds). *Textbook of Cultural Psychiatry*. Cambridge: Cambridge University Press, pp. 442–457.

Yakeley J, Johnston J, Adshead G, Allison L (2016). *Medical Psychotherapy*. Oxford: Oxford University Press.

Index

Tables, figures and boxes are indicated by an italic, *t*, *f* and *b* following the page number.

The manufacturer's authorised representative in the EU for product safety is Oxford University Press España S.A. of el Parque Empresarial San Fernando de Henares, Avenida de Castilla, 2 – 28830 Madrid (www.oup.es/en or product. safety@oup.com). OUP España S.A. also acts as importer into Spain of products made by the manufacturer.